An Atlas and Manual of

CORONARY INTRAVASCULAR
ULTRASOUND IMAGING

An Atlas and Manual of
CORONARY INTRAVASCULAR ULTRASOUND IMAGING

Paul Schoenhagen, MD, FAHA
and
Steven E. Nissen, MD, FACC

The Cleveland Clinic Foundation
Cleveland, Ohio

Associate Editors

E. Murat Tuzcu, MD, FACC
Anthony DeFranco, MD, FACC

Foreword by

Valentin Fuster
Mount Sinai Hospital, New York

The Parthenon Publishing Group
International Publishers in Medicine, Science & Technology

A CRC PRESS COMPANY
BOCA RATON   LONDON   NEW YORK   WASHINGTON, D.C.

Published in the USA by
The Parthenon Publishing Group Inc.
345 Park Avenue South, 10th Floor
New York
NY 10010
USA

Published in the UK and Europe by
The Parthenon Publishing Group
23–25 Blades Court
Deodar Road
London SW15 2NU
UK

Library of Congress Cataloging-in-Publication Data
Data available on application

British Library Cataloguing in Publication Data
Data available on application

ISBN 1-84214-274-7

First published in 2004

Composition by The Parthenon Publishing Group
Printed and bound by Butler & Tanner Ltd., Frome and London, UK

Contents

Acknowledgements

We wish to acknowledge the technicians in the Intravascular Ultrasound Core Laboratory: Tammy Churchill, Jennifer Coughlin, Deborah Hansen, Aaron Loyd, Cynthia Werle, Benlan Wong, Jay Zhitnik, clerical assistant Anthony Bebee, and our secretary Patricia Gooch.

List of contributing authors

Paul Schoenhagen, MD, FAHA
Departments of Diagnostic Radiology
Section of Cardiovascular Imaging and Department
    of Cardiovascular Medicine
The Cleveland Clinic Foundation

Steven E. Nissen, MD, FACC
Department of Cardiovascular Medicine
Medical Director
Cleveland Clinic Cardiovascular Coordinating
    Center
The Cleveland Clinic Foundation

E. Murat Tuzcu, MD, FACC
Professor of Medicine
and
Medical Director
Intravascular Ultrasound Core Laboratory
Department of Cardiovascular Medicine
The Cleveland Clinic Foundation

Anthony DeFranco, MD, FACC
Assistant Professor of Medicine
Michigan State University
and
Director, Heart and Vascular Center
Flint, Michigan

Richard D. White, MD, FACC
Department of Diagnostic Radiology and
    Cardiovascular Medicine
and
Clinical Director
Center for Integrated Non-Invasive Cardiovascular
    Imaging
The Cleveland Clinic Foundation

D. Geoffrey Vince, PhD
Department of Biomedical Engineering
Director, Vascular Wall Research
The Cleveland Clinic Foundation

Timothy Crowe, BS
Department of Cardiovascular Medicine
Technical Director
Intravascular Ultrasound and Angiography Core
    Laboratories
The Cleveland Clinic Foundation

Paula Shalling
Department of Cardiovascular Medicine
Systems Analyst
Intravascular Ultrasound and Angiography Core
    Laboratories
The Cleveland Clinic Foundation

William Magyar
Department of Cardiovascular Medicine
Senior Analyst
Intravascular Ultrasound Core Laboratory
The Cleveland Clinic Foundation

Editors' note

This book provides a systematic introduction to coronary imaging with intravascular ultrasound. It consists of two integrated parts, the Atlas and the Manual. Extensive cross-references between the two parts allow the reader either to review the Atlas and refer to the corresponding text paragraphs for additional information or to read the Manual and use the Atlas as traditional illustrations. The reference list and the subject index are connected to both, the Atlas and the Manual, allowing easy, rapid access to the information.

The style of the illustrations is uniform, showing a non-illustrated IVUS image together with an illustrated copy. The non-illustrated and illustrated images are either found in the same figure or, if several images are shown, in the subsequent figure.

Foreword

Historically, coronary angiography has represented the principal method used to characterize the extent and severity of coronary artery disease. Despite the nearly universal acceptance of angiography, this imaging modality is inherently limited in its ability to accurately describe the atherosclerotic disease process. An angiogram is merely a two-dimensional silhouette of the coronary lumen and cannot accurately portray the complex three-dimensional anatomy of the vessel wall. Accordingly, imaging techniques that directly visualize the arterial wall are achieving increasing importance in both research and the clinical assessment of atherosclerosis.

Newer imaging modalities such as intravascular ultrasound (IVUS) demonstrate that angiographic narrowings are only the focal manifestation of a diffuse, systemic disease process, which typically begins many years before symptoms occur. Importantly, sudden rupture or erosion of such mildly stenotic, but 'high-risk or vulnerable' lesions, causes most acute coronary syndromes. Rather than assessing luminal stenosis severity alone, modern atherosclerosis imaging is focused on plaque vulnerability and plaque burden. The rapidly accumulating data from these imaging modalities will undoubtedly open the way for more aggressive systemic treatments of atherosclerosis.

By combining the experience of an internationally recognized IVUS program with the innovative force of a leading imaging research center at the Cleveland Clinic, the Atlas provides a superb guide to IVUS and a visual description of current and future directions of atherosclerosis imaging. Although IVUS is an invasive approach to imaging the vessel wall, emerging non-invasive methods are developing rapidly. These include magnetic resonance imaging and computed tomography for the detection, quantification and serial observation of subclinical atherosclerosis. The insights provided by invasive methods such as IVUS and non-invasive emerging techniques are changing the way we think about atherosclerosis. These changes will revolutionize the assessment and management of patients with coronary artery disease.

The authors, Doctors Paul Schoenhagen and Steven Nissen, as well as the outstanding group of collaborators from the Cleveland Clinic, have to be congratulated for this *Atlas and Manual of Coronary Intravascular Ultrasound Imaging*. This is a unique compendium for 'prime time'.

Valentin Fuster, MD, PhD
Director, Wiener Cardiovascular Institute
and Kravis Center for Cardiovascular Health
Professor of Cardiology
Mount Sinai School of Medicine, New York, NY
Former President of the AHA
President Elect of the World Heart Federation

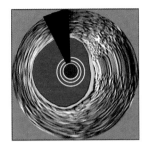

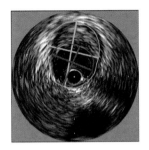

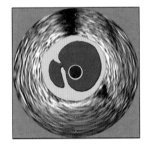

Section 1

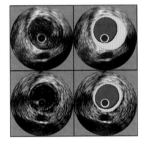

The Manual of
Coronary Intravascular
Ultrasound Imaging

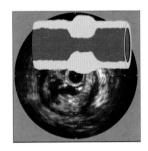

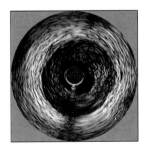

Introduction

Intravascular ultrasound (IVUS) is a tomographic imaging modality performed during coronary angiography. IVUS imaging allows the simultaneous assessment of lumen, vessel wall, and atherosclerotic plaque[1–10]. Therefore IVUS is complementary to selective coronary angiography, which is limited to a longitudinal silhouette of the lumen. When performed by an operator familiar with interventional, percutaneous techniques, the rate of complications during IVUS imaging is exceedingly low[11–13].

The experience with IVUS imaging has provided important insights into the anatomy of atherosclerotic lesion development. This information can guide patient management in different scenarios.

Clinical, interventional indications to perform IVUS are ambiguous angiographic findings and the guidance of percutaneous coronary intervention (PCI). In addition, IVUS has been established as the method of choice for the detection and serial observation of transplant vasculopathy and, more recently, for the serial observation of atherosclerotic plaque burden in atherosclerosis progression–regression trials.

This Manual describes the rationale, technique, and interpretation of IVUS imaging for diagnostic and therapeutic applications. The impact of ultrasound in understanding atherosclerotic coronary disease and its management is emphasized.

I

Principles of IVUS imaging

1.1 PRINCIPLES OF IVUS EXAMINATION (FIGURE 1)

IVUS is an invasive tomographic imaging modality[1,9,10]. During cardiac catheterization, an IVUS coronary catheter is advanced over a guide-wire beyond the target lesion (FIGURE 1). Subsequently, a pullback of the transducer tip through the lesion or segment of interest is performed. IVUS provides a series of tomographic, cross-sectional images of the vessel. Using a typical pullback speed of 0.5 mm/s and a frame-rate of 30 images/s, 60 images will be available from a pullback through a 1-mm segment. Typically, a subsample of these images is analyzed, depending on the clinical indication.

For the guidance of interventional procedures, the worst lesion site (where the luminal diameter is minimal, MLD) and a relatively normal, adjacent reference site is selected. In contrast, for volumetric analysis in research studies, multiple sequential IVUS images are obtained in a segment at constant intervals (FIGURE 1).

1.2 EQUIPMENT (FIGURES 2–4)

The equipment required to perform intracoronary ultrasound consists of three major components: a catheter incorporating a miniaturized ultrasound transducer, a pullback device, and a console containing the electronics necessary to reconstruct the image[1,9,10].

1.2.1 Catheter (FIGURES 2–4)

Current catheter sizes range from 2.6 to 3.5 French (0.87–1.17 mm). These catheters can be placed through a 6-French guiding catheter. The ultrasound transducer is mounted at the tip of the catheter. The ultrasound signal is produced in the transducer by passing an electrical current through the piezoelectric, crystalline material (usually a ceramic) that expands and contracts when electrically excited. After reflection from tissue, part of the ultrasound energy returns to the transducer and is converted into the image. High ultrasound frequencies are used, typically centered at 20–50 MHz (FIGURE 4). At 30 MHz, the wavelength is 50 µm, yielding a practical axial resolution of 150 µm. Lateral resolution, which depends on imaging depth, averages 250 µm for typical coronary diameters.

Two different transducer designs are commonly used: mechanically rotated devices and electronically switched multi-element array systems[9,10].

Mechanical systems

Mechanical probes use a drive cable to rotate a single transducer at the tip of the catheter at 1800 rpm (30 revolutions per second), sweeping an ultrasound beam perpendicular to the catheter. At approximately 1° increments, the transducer sends and receives ultrasound signals. The time delay and amplitude of these pulses provides 256 individual radial scan lines for each image. In mechanical catheter systems, the imaging transducer is located inside a protective sheath, which is advanced through the lesion or into the segment of interest. During the examination, the transducer is moved proximally and distally within the sheath, facilitating a smooth and uniform pullback. Mechanical catheters require flushing with saline to provide a fluid pathway for the ultrasound beam, because small air bubbles between the transducer and the protective sheath can degrade image quality.

Electronic systems

In electronic systems, multiple transducer elements (currently up to 64) arranged in an annular array are activated sequentially to generate the image. The array can be programmed so that one set of elements transmits while a second set receives simultaneously. The coordinated beam generated by groups of elements is known as a synthetic aperture array. The image can be manipulated to focus optimally at a broad range of depths. Currently available electronic systems can also provide simultaneous coloration of blood flow using the Doppler effect (FIGURE 20).

1.2.2 Pullback device (FIGURES 2 AND 3)

The transducer pullback can be performed either manually or using a motorized pullback device, which withdraws the catheter at a constant speed (between 0.25 and 1 mm/s, most frequently, 0.5 mm/s) (see Chapter 1.3.3)[9,10].

1.2.3 Imaging console (FIGURE 2)

The imaging console includes the hard- and software necessary to convert the IVUS signal to the image, the monitor and recording devices. Imaging studies are traditionally recorded on videotape, but newer systems permit digital recording and permanent archiving on a recordable CD-ROM.

1.3 EXAMINATION TECHNIQUE (FIGURE 1)

Standard interventional technique for intracoronary catheter delivery is used for intravascular ultrasound imaging[9,10]. Heparin and intracoronary nitroglycerin are routinely administered before the guidewire is inserted into the coronary artery. The operator then advances and retracts the imaging catheter over the wire, recording the images for subsequent analysis (FIGURE 1).

1.3.1 Safety of coronary ultrasound

The safety of intracoronary ultrasound is well documented[11-13]. Major complications, including dissection or vessel closure, are uncommon (less than < 0.5%) and typically occur in patients undergoing coronary intervention rather than diagnostic imaging

(FIGURES 92–95). Transient coronary spasm, which responds rapidly to intracoronary nitroglycerin, occurs in 1–3% of examinations. Transient ischemia, caused by introduction of the catheter in a small vessel or tight stenosis, is frequent in interventional procedures. Examination of vessels previously imaged by IVUS compared with non-instrumented vessels shows no accelerated progression of atheroma at 1 year of follow-up[13]. Despite this favorable safety profile, selective coronary instrumentation always carries a potential risk of significant vessel injury and should only be performed by operators experienced in diagnostic and interventional therapeutic intra-coronary catheter manipulation.

1.3.2 System setting (FIGURE 5)

System settings are very important in order to avoid misinterpretation of IVUS findings[9,10]. Gain refers to amplification of the returned signal. Increasing the overall gain can compensate for low catheter sensitivity, but at the expense of creating an image with increased noise and decreased gray-scale information (FIGURE 5). Time gain compensation (TGC) is a graduated adjustment of the signal gain, which is applied to balance the intensity of the image at different distances from the transducer.

1.3.3 Manual and motorized pullback
(FIGURES 1 AND 3)

As described above, the IVUS catheter is pulled through a vessel segment during continuous or intermittent imaging. The pullback is performed either manually or using a motorized pullback device[9,10]. The advantages of a manual transducer pullback are the ability to concentrate on specific regions of interest by pausing or slowing the transducer motion. Disadvantages include the possibility of skipping over significant pathology by pulling the transducer too quickly or unevenly. Motorized pullback devices withdraw the catheter at a constant speed of 0.25–1.0 mm/s (most frequently, 0.5 mm/s), allowing precise length and volume measurements.

In interrogating an aorto–ostial lesion of the left main coronary artery, it is important to disengage the guiding catheter from the ostium before the pull-back. Otherwise, the true aorto–ostial lumen may be masked by the guiding catheter and significant ostial lesions may be missed.

1.3.4 Cross-sectional, longitudinal, and three-dimensional display
(FIGURES 6 AND 7)

The standard displays of IVUS systems are cross-sectional individual images, reviewed individually and as a video sequence. Scrolling through adjacent cross-sectional images allows the experienced IVUS operator to obtain a three-dimensional impression of a vessel segment. Motorized transducer pullback and digital storage of cross-sectional images are necessary for longitudinal imaging (L-mode) (FIGURE 6). In an L-mode display, computerized image reconstruction techniques display a series of evenly spaced IVUS images along a single cut plane to approximate the longitudinal appearance of the artery[9,14]. Because the position of the IVUS catheter within the vessel varies along the pullback path, the cut plane should be selected through the center of the artery or lumen, rather than the center of the catheter. There are major limitations to the L-mode display, including the obligate straight reconstruction of the artery and the display of only a single cut plane. The changes of vessel size during the cardiac cycle result in a characteristic artifact described as the 'sawtooth' appearance (FIGURE 6). ECG-triggered image acquisition of image frames in the same cardiac phase can eliminate these artifacts[14].

Automated, three-dimensional reconstruction of IVUS data involves the use of advanced computer rendering techniques to display a shaded or wireframe image of the vessel, giving the operator a view of the vessel in its entirety[14-19] (FIGURE 7). However, true three-dimensional techniques require registration of the catheter path during the pullback. These methods are not yet included in current clinical systems but are an exciting area of research[19].

1.3.5 Radiofrequency–backscatter (FIGURE 8)

The raw IVUS signal is converted for conventional image presentation on the standard display. Additional analysis of the reflected ultrasound signal, analyzing several characteristics of the digitized ultrasound signal with integrated radiofrequency analysis, backscatter analysis, and elastography, allows advanced tissue characterization and more objective and reproducible methods of categorizing wall morphology and plaque components[20-26] (FIGURE 8). However, the clinical value of these advanced image analysis modalities is not completely defined[27].

1.3.6 Limitations of IVUS

Physical limitations of IVUS are the characteristic signal drop-out behind calcium, prohibiting the visualization of deep vessel structures (see Chapter 3.7). The physical size of ultrasound catheters (currently ≈ 1.0 mm) constitutes an important limitation in imaging severe stenoses and small vessels. In such vessels, the introduction of the catheter may cause dilatation of the vessel (Dotter effect) and may limit exact measurements[28]. The spatial resolution of IVUS ($> 150\,\mu m$) allows detailed analysis of vessel wall structures. However, important structures of atherosclerotic plaques, in particular the fibrous cap ($60–100\,\mu m$), cannot be reliably analyzed[29].

The invasive character of IVUS explains its preferential use in interventional cardiology and limits, in particular, the application in asymptomatic patients (Chapter 7). Therefore, the further development of non-invasive imaging modalities, including computed tomography and magnetic resonance imaging, will be important[29-31] (FIGURE 179).

2

Normal arterial anatomy by IVUS

In the IVUS image, the catheter is centered in the vessel, surrounded by the lumen, vessel wall and adjacent structures (FIGURE 9).

2.1 THE LUMEN (FIGURES 9–12)

At frequencies > 20 MHz, flowing blood exhibits a characteristic pattern of echogenicity, observed as finely textured echoes moving in a swirling pattern. This blood 'speckle' assists in image interpretation; it helps to differentiate the lumen and vessel wall (FIGURES 10 AND 11) and can confirm the communication between a dissection plane and the lumen (FIGURE 12). Blood speckle is more prominent at higher imaging frequencies, which may interfere with delineation of the blood–tissue interface (FIGURES 4 AND 11). Flushing of the vessel with saline or contrast during IVUS imaging can help to differentiate the lumen and vessel wall (FIGURES 10–12).

2.2 THE VESSEL WALL (FIGURE 9)

IVUS studies performed in excised, pressure-distended vessels have characterized the appearance of normal coronary arteries[5–8,32–36]. Ultrasound is reflected at tissue interfaces with an abrupt change in acoustic impedance. In the normal artery, two such interfaces are usually observed, one at the border between blood and the leading edge of the intima and the second at the external elastic membrane (EEM), which is located at the media–adventitia interface. The trailing edge of the intima is poorly defined and cannot be used reliably for measurements. The outer border of the adventitia is also indistinct, merging into the surrounding tissues. In good-quality images, the tunica media can sometimes be visualized as a distinct, relatively sonolucent layer (FIGURE 9)[36]. In young subjects, the normal value for intimal thickness is typically reported as 0.15 ± 0.07 mm. Most investigators use 0.25–0.50 mm as the upper limit of normal[32,36].

2.3 THE ADJACENT STRUCTURES (FIGURES 13–16)

Depending on the size of the artery, adjacent structures including arterial side-branches, cardiac veins, and the pericardium can be differentiated (FIGURE 13)[37]. During the pullback through the vessel, arterial side-branches characteristically appear at the periphery of the image and then join the imaged vessel (FIGURE 14). Cardiac veins run parallel to the artery or cross the artery, but characteristically do not join the imaged vessel. In addition, they can be differentiated by their systolic compression (FIGURES 15 AND 16). The adjacent structures are frequently used as landmarks to match images from serial examinations (see Chapter 7.3.1). However, the recognition may also be important in other situations. For example, in the recently described percutaneous *in situ* coronary artery bypass (PICAB) procedure, a conduit is created between a proximal coronary artery and a coronary vein, providing a new source of oxygenated blood to ischemic myocardium[38].

2.4 VESSEL BIFURCATION (FIGURE 17)

Because of unique hemodynamic properties, vessel bifurcations are predisposed to early and eccentric plaque development[39–44]. In IVUS images, the proximal segment of the side-branch can often be visualized during the pullback of the catheter through the main vessel. However, because of the eccentric position of the catheter relative to the side-branch, these images are difficult to evaluate. An example is the aorto–ostial bifurcation shown in Figure 17. The vessel wall of the aorta appears thickened and has different echogenicity, which may be an artifact secondary to oblique catheter position.

3

Image artifacts

Artifacts can adversely affect ultrasound images[45]. Some artifacts are related to the catheter design (mechanical vs. electronic systems), while others are unrelated to the system used.

3.1 GUIDE-WIRE ARTIFACT (FIGURE 18)

Using monorail catheter technology, the guide-wire lies outside the transducer and causes a typical artifact, which is characterized by a narrow-angled shadow (FIGURE 18). It is not recommended to retract the guide-wire during imaging in order to maintain secure access to the vessel.

3.2 RING-DOWN AND DIGITAL SUBTRACTION (FIGURES 19–21)

Ring-down artifacts are usually observed as bright halos of variable thickness surrounding the catheter (FIGURE 19)[45]. They are caused by acoustic oscillations in the transducer, which result in high-amplitude ultrasound signals that obscure the area immediately adjacent to the catheter. Ring-down artifacts create a zone of uncertainty adjacent to the transducer surface. Although time gain compensation (TGC) (Chapter 1.3.2) can be used to decrease this artifact, excessive ring-down suppression can reduce signals from true targets close to the catheter. In electronic systems, the transducers are surface-mounted, and ring-down is partially reduced by digital subtraction of a reference mask. If it is incorrectly performed, digital subtraction has the potential to remove real information or introduce false borders close to the transducer (FIGURES 20 AND 21).

3.3 NON-UNIFORM ROTATIONAL DISTORTION (FIGURE 22)

An important artifact, 'non-uniform rotational distortion' (NURD), arises from uneven drag on the drive cable of mechanical catheters, resulting in cyclical oscillations of rotational transducer speed, observed as visible distortion of the image[45]. NURD can occur for a number of reasons, including the presence of acute bends in the artery, tortuous guiding catheter shapes, kinking of the imaging sheath, or small lumen of the guiding catheter. A frequent and reversible cause is excessive tightening of the hemostatic valve.

3.4 SLOW FLOW (FIGURES 4, 10–12, 23)

The intensity of the blood speckle increases exponentially as blood flow velocity decreases. Therefore, flow stagnation, often most evident when the catheter is advanced across a tight stenosis, can limit the ability to differentiate lumen from echolucent tissue, including soft plaque, neointima, and thrombus. In these situations, flushing of the vessel with saline or contrast is particularly helpful for the differentiation of lumen and vessel wall (FIGURES 10–12).

3.5 CORONARY PULSATION AND MOTION ARTIFACT (FIGURES 24–26)

During the cardiac cycle, the IVUS transducer undergoes longitudinal displacement of as much as 5 mm in the axial direction and changes of angular orientation of the catheter relative to the vessel. In addition, the diameter of the coronary arteries undergoes characteristic changes during the cardiac cycle (FIGURE 24). In normal arteries, maximal vessel size is reached in systole but maximal flow is found in diastole, when the resistance to flow in the intramyocardial capillaries is minimal[46,47]. In contrast, at the site of muscle bridges, the artery size reaches a minimum diameter during systole, caused by the contraction of the muscle surrounding the vessel (FIGURE 25).

Because the image is reconstructed at 30 frames per second, occasionally part of an individual image is reconstructed from two subsequent frames, introducing false borders in such images (FIGURE 26). In general, careful analysis of IVUS images always includes a review of adjacent images in order to recognize this and other artifacts.

3.6 CATHETER OBLIQUITY, ECCENTRICITY (FIGURE 17)

Geometric distortion can result from imaging in an oblique plane (not perpendicular to the long axis of the vessel). Current image reconstruction techniques assume that the vessel is circular, and that the catheter is located in the center of the artery and parallel to the long axis of the vessel. However, in clinical practice, this is often not the case and both transducer obliquity and vessel curvature can introduce an elliptical image distortion. Transducer obliquity is especially important in large vessels and can result in an overestimation of dimensions and a reduction in image quality[48]. The latter phenomenon occurs because the amplitude of the echo reflected from an interface depends on the angle at which the beam strikes the interface. The strongest signals are obtained when the catheter is coaxial within the vessel and when the beam strikes the target at a 90° angle. If the IVUS beam strikes the wall of the vessel in a shallow angle, image quality deteriorates. An example is shown in Figure 17. Because of the eccentric catheter position at the ostium, the wall of the aorto–ostial segment appears thickened with low echogenicity.

3.7 CALCIUM SHADOW
(FIGURES 27 AND 46)

Calcium is an important part of atherosclerotic plaques and IVUS has a high sensitivity in its detection[49,50]. However, almost all IVUS energy is reflected by calcium, causing a characteristic signal drop-out or multiple reflections of concentric arcs behind the calcified tissue (FIGURES 27 AND 46) (see Chapter 5.2.3).

4

IVUS measurements

Borders between tissue with different composition and acoustic properties cause strong ultrasound reflection. Two such borders in the coronary artery wall are the lumen/intimal border and the external elastic membrane (EEM)[5,6,35,36]. The strong signal originating at these tissue interfaces allows recognition and manual or automated planimetry. Distance and area measurements are subsequently derived from planimetry. Details of recommended measurements have been reported in current clinical AHA/ACC and ESC guidelines[9,10].

4.1 LUMEN MEASUREMENTS
(FIGURES 28 AND 29)

Once the lumen border has been delineated, the following lumen measurements are derived. All measurements are performed relative to the center of the lumen, rather than relative to the center of the IVUS catheter.

Lumen cross-sectional area (CSA): the area bound by the luminal border.

Minimum and maximum lumen diameters: the shortest and longest diameters through the center point of the lumen, respectively.

Lumen eccentricity: calculated as 100 x [(maximum lumen diameter - minimum lumen diameter) divided by maximum lumen diameter].

Lumen area stenosis: calculated as [(reference lumen CSA - minimum lumen CSA)/reference lumen CSA]. The reference segment used should be specified (proximal, distal, largest, or average). This measurement is similar to the angiographic percentage stenosis.

Caveats

Comparison of luminal measurements between IVUS and angiography usually shows a close correlation for vessels without atherosclerosis. However, for diseased arteries, investigators report only a moderate correlation ($r = 0.7$–0.8) and a standard error > 0.5 mm[8,51]. Comparative studies show the greatest disparities between angiography and ultrasound after mechanical interventions[52]. In this setting, the shape of the lumen may be extremely complex, with plaque fissures or deep wall dissections[53]. These extraluminal channels contribute little to blood flow, and are therefore typically not included when tracing the luminal contour. A commonly applied approach distinguishes the true lumen area from the 'dissection area'.

4.2 EEM MEASUREMENTS
(FIGURES 28 AND 29)

After delineation of the EEM border, the following measurements are derived:

EEM cross-sectional area (CSA): the area bounded by the EEM border

Minimum and maximum EEM diameters: the shortest and longest diameters through the center point of the EEM area, respectively.

Caveats

A discrete interface at the outer border between the media and the adventitia is almost invariably present within IVUS images and corresponds closely to the location of the EEM[5,6,35,36]. The recommended term for this measurement is EEM area, rather than the alternative term 'vessel area'. External elastic membrane circumference and area cannot be measured reliably at sites where large side-branches originate or in the setting of extensive calcification, because of acoustic shadowing (FIGURE 27). If acoustic shadowing involves a relatively small arc (< 90°), planimetry of the circumference can be performed by extrapolation from the closest identifiable EEM border, although measurement accuracy and reproducibility will be reduced. If the circumferential extent of a calcification is more than 90°, EEM measurements should not be reported. Similarly, some stent designs may obscure the EEM border and render measurements unreliable.

4.3 PLAQUE (ATHEROMA) MEASUREMENTS (FIGURES 28–30)

Plaque area measurements are derived by subtracting lumen area from EEM area (FIGURE 28).

Plaque cross-sectional area (CSA): the EEM CSA minus the lumen CSA

Maximum and minimum plaque thicknesses: the largest and shortest distances from the intimal leading edge to the EEM border along any line passing through the center of the lumen.

Circumferential extent of disease is commonly classified by determining whether abnormal intimal thickening is present throughout the 360° arterial circumference. Based on these observations, plaque eccentricity is defined as:

Plaque eccentricity: 100 x [(maximum plaque thickness - minimum plaque thickness)/maximum plaque thickness].

Plaque burden: atheroma CSA divided by EEM CSA. The atheroma burden represents the area within the EEM occupied by atheroma, regardless of the lumen compromise.

The *longitudinal extent* of disease is defined as 'diffuse' if the intimal thickness is abnormal at every site within the segment, or as focal if sites adjacent to the lesion site have minimal disease.

Caveats

Because the leading edge of the media (the internal elastic membrane) is not well delineated, IVUS measurements cannot determine the true

histological atheroma area (the area bounded by the internal elastic membrane)[7]. Accordingly, IVUS studies use the EEM and lumen CSA measurements to calculate a surrogate for true atheroma area, the 'plaque plus media area'[9,10]. In histological studies, early atherosclerotic lesions are associated with structural changes in media thickness[54]. However, in clinical practice, the inclusion of the media into the atheroma area does not constitute a major limitation of IVUS because the media represents only a very small fraction of the atheroma CSA. Plaque area measurements performed in this fashion correlate closely with histology[33–35,46].

It is important to differentiate plaque burden, which is the percentage of the EEM area occupied by atheroma at the lesion site, and angiographic percentage stenosis, which represents an expression of luminal narrowing at the lesion relative to a reference segment.

4.4 CALCIUM MEASUREMENTS (FIGURES 27 AND 46)

IVUS is a very sensitive *in vivo* method for the detection of coronary calcium, which is a indicator of atherosclerotic plaque[49,50]. Calcified deposits appear as bright echoes that obstruct the penetration of ultrasound, a phenomenon known as 'acoustic shadowing'. Therefore, IVUS can detect only the leading edge of calcified plaque but cannot determine its thickness.

Calcium deposits are described qualitatively according to their location and distribution:

Superficial or deep: the leading edge of the acoustic shadowing appears within the superficial or deep 50% of the atheroma thickness, respectively.

The *arc of calcium* can be measured (in degrees) by using an electronic protractor centered on the lumen.

The *length of the calcified deposit* in a coronary segment can be measured using motorized transducer pullback.

4.5 REMODELING MEASUREMENTS (FIGURE 31, SEE CHAPTER 5.1.2)

Arterial remodeling refers to the changes in EEM area that occur during the development of atherosclerotic lesions[55]. IVUS imaging allows *in vivo* assessment of vascular remodeling[56–65].

An index or ratio that describes the magnitude and direction of remodeling is expressed as lesion EEM CSA/reference EEM CSA. Expansive (positive) and constrictive (negative) remodeling are defined as a lesion EEM area greater or smaller than the reference EEM area, respectively. A number of dichotomous definitions of remodeling have been proposed based on a comparison with either the proximal reference, distal reference, or both[57–65]. A common definition compares lesion site and proximal reference and defines expansive (positive) and constrictive (negative) remodeling as a ratio of > 1.05 and < 0.95[59,64].

4.6 STENT MEASUREMENTS
(FIGURES 32–34)

The stent adds another border to the IVUS image. The following measurements are commonly reported:

Stent CSA: the area bounded by the stent struts.

Minimum and maximum stent diameters: the shortest and longest diameters through the center of the stent, respectively.

Stent symmetry: 100 x [(maximum stent diameter - minimum stent diameter)/maximum stent diameter].

Stent expansion: the minimum stent CSA compared with a reference area, which can be the proximal, distal, largest, or average reference area.

Strut apposition refers to the proximity of stent struts to the arterial wall[66,67]. Good apposition is defined as sufficiently close contact to preclude blood flow between any strut and the underlying wall. Documentation of apposition can be enhanced by flushing saline or contrast from the guiding catheter to confirm the presence or absence of flow behind the struts.

Caveats

Metallic stent struts are strong reflectors of ultrasound and therefore appear as echogenic points or arcs along the circumference of the vessel. Depending on the design and material, each stent has a slightly different appearance. Slotted-tube or multi-cellular stents appear as focal metallic points, whereas coiled stents appear as arcs of metal that subtend small sections of the vessel wall. Similar to the calcium shadow (Chapter 3.7), there is an area of

signal drop-out behind the stent struts (FIGURES 90 AND 99). Recently introduced covered stents (plastic membrane) cause signal attenuation and have a particular appearance on IVUS (FIGURE 33).

4.7 LENGTH MEASUREMENTS (FIGURE 6)

Length measurements using IVUS can be derived from images obtained using motorized transducer pullbacks (number of seconds x pullback speed). This approach can be used to determine the length of a lesion, but also specific longitudinal features including the length of calcifications. A more practical approach is to obtain length measurements using the L-mode display. However, the missing information about vessel curvature in the straight L-mode display is a significant limitation (Chapter 1.3.4).

4.8 VOLUMETRIC MEASUREMENTS
(FIGURES 35,128,129)

For quantitative volumetric IVUS analysis, a segment of interest is selected between two characteristic fiduciary points (start- and end-point, e.g. side-branches). Starting at the distal fiduciary location, single frames are selected from the digitized pullback sequence at 0.5–1-mm intervals[68,69]. For each of the selected frames, the lumen and EEM cross-sectional areas are measured. The Simpson rule is applied to calculate plaque volume by multiplying plaque area and distance between adjacent images. An alternative approach is the ECG-gated selection of frames in pre-defined relation to the cardiac cycle[19,70,71]. Side-branches and calcium are limitations of these volumetric approaches because the EEM area cannot be measured reliably at these sites. The following guidelines have been proposed:

When side-branches are encountered at one of the selected frames, the EEM border measurements are extrapolated, but the intimal leading edge measurements are not. If calcification leads to acoustic shadowing involving a relatively small arc (< 90°), planimetry of the circumference can be performed by extrapolation from the closest identifiable EEM border, although measurement accuracy and reproducibility will be reduced. If the circumferential extent of a calcification is more than 90°, EEM measurements should not be reported. In studies examining in-stent restenosis, the volumetric analysis of the neointimal tissue is the primary end-point. Because most stent designs obscure the EEM border, total plaque volume is typically not reported in these studies[72,73].

5

Plaque (atheroma) morphology

5.1 GEOMETRY (FIGURES 36–44)

Plaque geometry describes the form and distribution of atherosclerotic lesions. Important and interrelated characteristics are plaque size, stenosis severity, longitudinal extent of the lesion (diffuse versus focal), circumferential extent of the stenosis (eccentric versus concentric), and extent and direction of arterial remodeling. Concomitant changes of these characteristics explain the frequent dissociation between angiography and IVUS findings and may also have a relationship to plaque stability[74].

5.1.1 Plaque size and relationship to luminal stenosis (FIGURE 36)

A direct comparison between IVUS and angiography demonstrates that the extent and severity of disease as visualized by angiography and ultrasound are frequently discrepant[74]. IVUS studies demonstrate that there is no close relationship between the size of the atheroma and the size of the lumen. This phenomenon is a consequence of two major factors, the diffuse nature of atherosclerosis affecting the angiographically 'normal reference sites'[75] and adaptive enlargement of the EEM (remodeling), which maintains lumen size despite plaque progression[55].

5.1.2 Arterial remodeling (FIGURES 37–42)

Arterial remodeling in human coronary arteries was initially described in a postmortem study by Glagov and colleagues. They found a positive correlation between EEM and atheroma area[55]. At lesions with a percentage stenosis < 40%, plaque accumulation was accommodated by an increase in arterial size, resulting in a stable lumen area (FIGURE 38). In more advanced lesions, remodeling was less evident and plaque progression was associated with luminal stenosis. The authors hypothesized that this phenomenon represented a compensatory mechanism to preserve lumen size. Subsequent IVUS studies allowed the *in vivo* investigation of remodeling and confirmed the correlation between EEM and plaque area (FIGURES 37–39, 41)[57,58]. Subsequent IVUS studies demonstrated that, at certain diseased sites, the EEM may actually shrink, contributing to luminal stenosis. This process is called constrictive (negative) remodeling or arterial shrinkage (FIGURES 37, 40, 42)[59,60]. Constrictive remodeling has a particularly prominent role in restenosis after mechanical intervention[60–63].

Recently, several IVUS studies have examined the relationship between remodeling and clinical presentation in patients with coronary artery disease[64,65]. Expansive (positive) remodeling is significantly more prevalent in patients with unstable coronary presentation, and constrictive (negative) remodeling more prevalent in patients with stable coronary syndromes. Based on these results, it has been hypothesized that arterial remodeling is related to plaque vulnerability (see Chapter 7.1).

In order to avoid misunderstandings, it has therefore been suggested that the terms 'positive' and 'negative' remodeling should be replaced with 'expansive' and 'constrictive' remodeling.

5.1.3 Eccentricity (FIGURE 43)

The circumferential distribution of the atheroma is described by its eccentricity (see Chapter 4.3). Early lesions and lesions at vessel bifurcations are characterized by eccentric distribution and suggest a relationship between local flow hemodynamics and lesion development[39-44].

5.1.4 Diffuse disease (FIGURE 44)

The strength of coronary angiography is the precise description of *focal*, severe luminal stenoses. However, it is well known that the atherosclerotic disease process is more diffuse, and this is frequently reflected in angiographic 'mild luminal irregularities'. The comparison with IVUS has confirmed the diffuse character of coronary artery disease. It is difficult to describe the longitudinal extent of disease burden and there are currently no clear guidelines. An emerging approach is the description of plaque volumes in entire vessel segments (see Chapters 4.8 and 7.2).

5.2 PLAQUE ECHOGENICITY (FIGURES 45–49)

Ultrasound provides information about the morphology of atherosclerotic plaques *in vivo*. However, IVUS is limited in the characterization of specific histological contents. Studies have compared the ultrasound appearance of plaques to histology in freshly explanted human arteries[33-35,76,77]. Lipid-rich lesions generate low-intensity hypoechoic echoes (FIGURE 45). Frequently, these lesions exhibit a prominent echogenic border structure at the lumen–intima interface. This may correspond to the anatomic structure of the fibrous cap. However, it should be emphasised that the fibrous cap of most unstable lesions is too thin to be resolved by IVUS (< 50 μm). Fibrous or calcified tissues are relatively echogenic (FIGURE 45). Calcium obstructs ultrasound penetration and therefore creates a characteristic signal void (acoustic shadowing), which obscures the underlying vessel wall (FIGURES 45 AND 46).

Although contemporary IVUS systems produce detailed views of the vessel wall, standard interpretation relies on simple visual inspection of acoustic reflections to determine plaque composition. The textures of different tissue components may exhibit comparable acoustic properties and therefore appear quite similar by IVUS. For example, an echolucent luminal mass of tissue may represent intracoronary thrombus or an atheroma with a high lipid content (FIGURES 49–52). Thus, IVUS is not consistently able to predict plaque components in comparison to histology[76-78]. More objective and automated classification of atheromatous lesions is possible with advanced ultrasound data analysis. Radiofrequency analysis and elastography have been validated in *ex vivo* studies against histology and are emerging for clinical application (see Chapter 1.3.5) (FIGURE 8)[20-27].

5.2.1 Echolucent plaques (FIGURE 45)

The low echogenicity of these plaques is generally the result of high lipid content in a mostly cellular lesion[33,79]. However, a zone of reduced echogenicity may also be attributable to a necrotic zone within the plaque, an intramural hemorrhage, or a thrombus. The term 'soft' plaque should be avoided because the echodensity does not refer to the plaque's structural, mechanical characteristics.

5.2.2 Echodense plaques (FIGURE 45)

These plaques have an intermediate echogenicity between echolucent atheromas and highly echogenic calcific plaques and, together with mixed lesions, represent the majority of atherosclerotic lesions. In histological studies, a correlation between echodensity and plaque fibrosis has been described. However, very dense fibrous plaques may produce sufficient attenuation and acoustic shadowing to be misclassified as calcified by IVUS.

5.2.3 Calcified plaque (FIGURES 45 AND 46)

Ultrasound imaging has shown significantly higher sensitivity than fluoroscopy in the detection of coronary calcification[49,50]. The significance of coronary calcifications is complex and, in particular, their relation to plaque stability is unclear. Large calcification may in fact be associated with lesion stability. In contrast, microcalcifications are frequently found in lipid-rich necrotic core areas of unstable plaques and may not be well reflected in IVUS images[80,81].

5.2.4 Mixed plaque (FIGURES 47 AND 48)

Coronary plaques frequently contain tissue components with different acoustic characteristics. In these 'mixed' plaques, areas with various morphology are seen within individual cross-sectional images or in adjacent cross-sections (FIGURES 44, 47, 48, 102). In these mixed lesions, further classification of plaque components may be possible with advance image analysis, including radiofrequency analysis (FIGURE 8)[22,26].

5.2.5 Thrombus (FIGURES 49–52)

By IVUS, a thrombus is usually recognized as an intraluminal mass, often with a layered, lobulated, or pedunculated appearance. Thrombi may appear relatively echolucent or have a more variable echogenicity, with speckling or scintillation. Blood flow in 'microchannels' may also be apparent within some thrombi (FIGURES 67–70). Stagnant blood flow can simulate a thrombus, with a grayish-white accumulation of specular echoes within the vascular lumen (FIGURE 23). Injection of contrast or saline may disperse the stagnant flow and allow differentiation of stasis from thrombosis (FIGURE 11). None of these morphological features is pathognomonic for thrombus, and IVUS is unreliable in differentiating acute thrombi from echolucent plaques because of the similar echogenicities of lipid-rich tissue, loose connective tissue, stagnant blood and thrombi[82]. This has important clinical consequences for patients presenting with acute coronary syndromes, because, in the presence of a ruptured plaque with superimposed acute thrombosis and additional lesions, the accurate identification of the 'culprit' lesion may not always be possible.

5.2.6 Intimal hyperplasia (FIGURES 34 AND 101)

The histological composition of the neointimal tissue after PCI is complex. Recent studies suggest that both cell proliferation and enhanced extracellular matrix (ECM) accumulation contribute to in-stent restenosis, and that their relative importance changes over time[83]. This may be reflected in the ultrasound appearance. The intimal hyperplastic tissue characteristic of early in-stent restenosis often has a very low echogenicity, at times less echogenic than the blood speckle in the lumen. Appropriate system settings are critical to avoid suppressing this relative non-echogenic material. The intimal hyperplasia of late in-stent restenosis often appears more echogenic.

5.2.7 Coronary venous bypass grafts
(FIGURE 53)

In vein grafts, wall morphology and plaque characteristics are different from those in native coronary arteries. The wall of the bypass graft is free from the surrounding tissue and has no side-branches. *In situ* vein grafts do not have an EEM. However, vein grafts typically undergo 'arterialization', with morphological changes that include intimal fibrous thickening, medial hypertrophy, and lipid deposition. The 'EEM area' is measured by tracing the outer border of the sonolucent zone, which typically follows the intima. All other measurements, including atheroma area and plaque burden, are calculated in a similar fashion to those for native coronary disease.

5.2.8 Unstable ('vulnerable') high-risk lesion, plaque ulceration and rupture
(FIGURES 54–65)

Most acute coronary syndromes are caused by sudden rupture or erosion of vulnerable plaques[84]. Plaque vulnerability is defined prospectively as the tendency of a lesion to rupture or erode, causing subsequent thrombosis. IVUS can identify plaque rupture but is limited in the identification of vulnerable lesions before rupture/erosion[85]. Plaque rupture or ulceration is defined by IVUS as a cavity in the vessel wall with disruption of the intima and flow observed within the plaque cavity (FIGURES 54–65). Features supporting intimal disruption are an irregular intimal surface of ulcerated plaques and visible torn edges in video sequences. Blood flow in the vessel wall cavity is an important criterion, and contrast injections may be used to prove and define the communication point[9,10,86,87]. However, ruptured plaques may have a highly variable appearance by IVUS, in particular in the presence of a superimposed thrombus (see Chapter 5.2.5).

Ultrasound studies have found an association between echolucent, presumably lipid-laden, plaques and acute coronary syndromes[88–91]. In addition, expansive (positive) remodeling is consistently observed in culprit lesions causing unstable clinical presentation[64,65,92–96]. Recently, the term high-risk plaque (HRP) has been suggested for a lesion with imaging features as described above. This term acknowledges the limitations of *in vivo* imaging for the *prospective* identification of plaques at risk to rupture and cause acute coronary syndromes (vulnerable plaques)[29,85].

5.2.9 Other lesion morphology

(FIGURES 66–71)

A true aneurysm is defined as an expansion of the vessel at a lesion site that includes all layers of the vessel wall (FIGURE 66). Frequently, clinical definitions require that the EEM and lumen diameter are at least 50% larger than the proximal reference segment. Positive arterial remodeling and focal aneurysms may be extremes on a spectrum of a common pathophysiological process[97]. A pseudo-aneurysm is defined as a disruption of the EEM, usually observed after intervention (FIGURES 99 AND 100).

It is sometimes difficult to differentiate true versus false lumen (FIGURES 67–70). Possible hints are that a true lumen is surrounded by intima, media, and adventitia.

The IVUS literature about non-atherosclerotic wall thickening is limited[98]. Figure 71 shows images of a young patient with documented Takayasu arteritis involving the aorta, documented by histology. Thickening of the coronary artery wall was previously documented with IVUS but histological diagnosis of the coronary involvement was not available.

6

Established clinical applications

6.1 ASSESSMENT OF ANGIOGRAPHICALLY INDETERMINATE LESIONS
(FIGURES 72–82)

Angiographically normal coronary arteries are encountered in 10–15% of patients undergoing catheterization for suspected coronary disease. IVUS commonly detects occult disease in these patients[99,100]. Certain lesion subsets elude accurate angiographic characterization, despite thorough examination using multiple radiographic projections. These angiographically ambiguous lesions include intermediate lesions of uncertain stenotic severity (FIGURES 72–81), aneurysmal lesions (FIGURE 66), ostial stenosis (FIGURE 82), disease at branching sites, tortuous vessels, left main stem lesions (see Chapter 6.1.1) (FIGURE 82), sites with focal spasm, sites with plaque rupture, morphology after coronary angioplasty (FIGURES 77–79), intraluminal filling defects/thrombus, and angiographically hazy lesions[101].

IVUS is frequently employed to examine lesions with the above characteristics, in some cases providing additional evidence useful in determining whether the stenosis is clinically significant[102,103]. Depending on the clinical scenario, it may be preferable to obtain intracoronary hemodynamic information, for example, an assessment of fractional flow reserve rather than anatomic information.

6.1.1 Left main coronary artery
(FIGURES 80–82)

Assessment of left main (LM) disease by angiography represents a particularly difficult clinical problem (FIGURES 80–82)[104–106]. Aortic cusp opacification or 'streaming' of contrast may obscure the ostium, the short length of the vessel may leave no normal segment for comparison, and the distal left main artery may be concealed by the left anterior descending coronary artery/left circumflex coronary artery (LAD/LCX) bifurcation (FIGURES 80 AND 81). In these situations, ultrasound often can provide additional information. The pullback is performed with the guiding catheter disengaged from the LM ostium. There is currently no consensus regarding the cross-sectional area at which the left main obstruction is considered critical. However, an absolute area $< 9\,mm^2$ has been proposed as a criterion for left main stenosis severity requiring revascularization. Importantly, IVUS has demonstrated physiological, non-atherosclerotic ostial LM narrowing (FIGURE 82)[106].

6.2 ASSESSMENT OF TRANSPLANT VASCULOPATHY (FIGURE 83)

Coronary transplant vasculopathy represents the major cause of death after the first year following cardiac transplantation. Its development is often clinically silent because the transplanted heart is denervated and ischemia is usually not detected with functional testing until the disease is advanced[107–109]. Surveillance angiography identifies focal, stenotic disease in 10–20% of patients at 1 year and 50% by 5 years[110,111]. However, it underestimates the diffuse nature of transplant vasculopathy with early intimal thickening[112]. IVUS allows the assessment of early plaque accumulation before luminal stenosis develops. Using $> 0.5\,mm$ as a threshold for intimal thickening, the prevalence of arteriopathy detected by ultrasound is 50% by 1 year[113-116]. Therefore, IVUS has emerged as the preferred method for early detection[117-122]. Ultrasound studies have demonstrated an association between the severity of transplant vasculopathy and clinical outcome, with an increased incidence of death, myocardial infarction or re-transplantation in those with more severe disease[118-120].

The intimal thickening of the coronary arteries that develops after cardiac transplantation must be differentiated from donor transmitted atherosclerotic coronary disease. Surprisingly, despite the young age and non-cardiac cause of death of heart donors, conventional atherosclerosis is frequently present in donor hearts at the time of transplantation. In a study from our group, atherosclerotic lesions were detected in 56% of patients at a mean donor age of 32 years[121]. However, the natural history of these 'donor lesions' after transplantation is largely unknown[122].

Important information has been gained from serial IVUS studies after cardiac transplantation. IVUS protocols use a variety of sampling approaches for the detection and surveillance of transplant vasculopathy. Serial intravascular imaging has been used to evaluate therapies for transplant vasculopathy, including immunosuppressive medications, statin drugs, and angiotensin-converting enzyme (ACE) inhibitors. In these studies, IVUS images are compared at baseline and follow-up. Individual images are often compared side by side, with angiographic and IVUS landmarks (side-branches, pericardium, and cardiac veins) used to match sites. These focal approaches include the examination of three or four sites at least 1 cm apart, or the selection using predefined criteria typically including the site with most severe intimal thickening. Rapidly progressive intimal thickening (0.5 mm increase) in the first year after transplantation has been shown to have negative prognostic significance[123].

Volumetric approaches use an automated pullback between two fiduciary points to determine the entire volume of the EEM, lumen, and intima (see Chapter 4.8). Volumetric analysis of entire segments has developed into the preferred method because of its minimal variability. Using serial, volumetric analysis, a recent study has demonstrated attenuated intimal hyperplasia during treatment with a rapamycin-containing immunosuppressive regimen in comparison to the standard regimen[124]. This was associated with a reduction in clinical events, suggesting the possible use of plaque burden as a

surrogate end-point in pharmacological studies (Chapter 7.2).

It remains to be seen whether non-invasive imaging techniques, in particular computer tomography (CT) and magnetic resonance imaging (MRI) can provide sufficient detailed information to allow the serial assessment of transplant vasculopathy[125,126].

6.3 INTERVENTIONAL APPLICATIONS
(FIGURES 84–101)

Although IVUS has played a pivotal role in understanding the effects of interventional devices, the precise clinical role for intravascular ultrasound during intervention has not been well defined in large-scale clinical trials. It would be beyond the scope of this Manual to discuss specific interventional indications. However, the principles and pertinent literature will be summarized.

6.3.1 Pre-interventional target lesion assessment (FIGURES 84–89)

Pre-interventional IVUS is used to analyze the target lesion and select the interventional approach most suitable for a specific lesion. Several plaque characteristics, including measurements of atheroma severity, plaque distribution, depth and extent of calcification, arterial remodeling, and the presence of thrombi or dissections can affect the decision to use a particular device. Single-center studies have reported that ultrasound imaging often influences the operators' appreciation of target lesions and the optimal approach to therapy[102,103]. More recent studies describe that pre-interventional plaque characteristics, including echogenicity and remodeling, determine target lesion revascularization rate (TVR) during follow-up after PCI[88–90,127–129].

6.3.2 Guidance for angioplasty and atherectomy

Based on angiographic observations, plaque compression was originally suggested as an important mechanism for lumen gain after balloon angioplasty. However, direct examination of the plaque before and after interventions with IVUS demonstrated that 'axial redistribution' and vessel wall stretching, rather than compression of the plaque, are the major mechanisms of lumen gain post-procedure[130–134]. The frequency of plaque fracture and arterial wall dissection after PCI was much higher than suggested by angiography, with evidence of disruption seen in about 50% and 75% of cases, respectively[51–53,134].

Several studies examined whether post-interventional morphological features, such as the presence or extent of dissection, lumen size, or plaque burden, are related to restenosis rate. Some studies identified residual plaque burden as an independent predictor of outcome, but the results are conflicting[135–137]. IVUS criteria have been used to guide balloon angioplasty, typically allowing larger balloon size[138–140]. However, the long-term clinical impact has not been established.

IVUS can facilitate lesion selection for directional coronary atherectomy, because the presence of significant calcification is an important predictor of procedural failure[141]. A consistent finding from IVUS studies of directional atherectomy is the substantial residual plaque burden after atherectomy despite excellent angiographic result[141]. Several studies have addressed the issue of more aggressive plaque removal on the basis of ultrasound imaging, but the results are conflicting[142–145].

IVUS imaging in the context of high-speed rotational atherectomy has confirmed the principle of differential cutting with selective removal of less compliant plaque material, most notably calcium[146]. Measurement of the true vessel size by ultrasound may allow safe use of larger burrs, with a greater lumen gain and less residual plaque burden[147]. As in the case of directional atherectomy, IVUS demonstrates a large residual plaque burden after rotablation.

6.3.3 Guidance for stenting
(FIGURE 90)

IVUS imaging has played a pivotal role in understanding and optimizing the benefits of coronary stent therapy. Columbo and colleagues[148] demonstrated that deployment with conventional balloon pressures resulted in a high incidence of incomplete stent expansion and apposition (FIGURE 90). Ultrasound imaging to guide high-pressure dilatation achieved full expansion and complete stent apposition in a large percentage of patients, allowing the use of a simplified anti-thrombotic regimen of aspirin and ticlopidine without warfarin. These results established high-pressure stent implantation, and larger trials confirmed the safety of stent implantation without IVUS guidance using high pressures and antiplatelet therapy alone[149–151].

Several studies have directly addressed the question of whether the increased lumen areas resulting from ultrasound guidance lead to a significant reduction in restenosis[152–154]. These studies demonstrate a reduction in revascularization but not in the incidence of myocardial infarction or mortality.

There is currently no consensus regarding optimal ultrasound procedural end-points for stent implantation. While most operators advocate complete apposition of the stent struts to the wall, the extent of stent expansion in comparison to the reference required for optimal results remains controversial. Suggested relative stent expansion criteria, which compare the minimal stent area to that of reference segments, include 90% or 100% of the distal and 80% or 90% of the average reference lumen areas[154].

6.3.4 Dissection, intramural hematoma and other complications after intervention
(FIGURES 91–100)

IVUS is commonly employed to detect and direct the treatment of dissection and other complications after intervention (FIGURES 91–100)[51–53,134,152]. A classification of dissections according to their depth has been proposed with intimal, medial, and adventitial extension. Separation of neointimal tissue inside the stent struts is occasionally seen after treatment of in-stent restenosis.

An intramural hematoma (FIGURE 98) is defined as an accumulation of blood within the medial space, displacing the internal elastic membrane inward and EEM outward[9].

6.3.5 The restenotic lesion and in-stent restenosis (FIGURES 34 AND 101)

Ultrasound studies in peripheral vessels by Pasterkamp and colleagues[59] provided the first evidence that constrictive (negative) remodeling, or localized shrinkage of the vessel, was a major mechanism of late lumen loss after PCI in addition to intimal proliferation. In a serial study by Mintz and colleagues[60] >70% of lumen loss after PTCA was attributable to the decrease in EEM area, whereas growth of the neointimal area accounted for only 23% of the loss.

Unlike this restenotic response after angioplasty or atherectomy, which is a mixture of constrictive (negative) arterial remodeling and neointimal growth, in-stent restenosis is primarily due to neointimal proliferation (FIGURE 101). In serial IVUS studies of stented coronary segments, no significant change occurred in the area bound by stent struts, indicating that stents can resist the arterial remodeling process[156,157]. Subsequent studies demonstrated that late lumen loss correlated strongly with the degree of in-stent neointimal growth $(r = 0.98)$[73,158,159]. Because the degree of in-stent neointimal hyperplasia is independent of the achieved stent lumen size, restenosis decreases as a function of increasing absolute post-procedure minimal stent area[160,161]. This explains the higher restenosis rates in smaller vessels and inadequately expanded stents, in which the acute lumen gain does not accommodate tissue proliferation during follow-up.

In most of the above-cited serial imaging studies, the restenotic process was assessed by first identifying the image slice with the smallest lumen area at follow-up and subsequently matching of the same image slice on the pre-intervention or post-intervention study. Such serial stent studies are limited by the fact that the axial position of the restenotic lesion is usually different from the smallest pre-intervention or post-intervention target site. More recently, volumetric analysis of an entire arterial segment rather than the worst lesion site alone has been used. This approach can determine whether the site of maximum tissue growth has occurred within the stent or in the adjacent reference segment near the stent border[72,73,161].

Volumetric IVUS analysis of the stented segment is a particularly attractive approach in understanding the effects of radiation therapy (brachytherapy)[162], and drug-eluting stents[163,164].

6.3.6 Brachytherapy and drug-eluting stents

Ultrasound has been useful in refining the technique of brachytherapy[162,165]. IVUS studies have demonstrated that radiation has the potential to profoundly inhibit neointimal proliferation within a stent, but also to accelerate restenosis at the edges of the treatment region, where the dosing falls off ('candy wrapper' effect)[166]. Dose distribution is dependent on the thickness and composition of the atheroma and the position of the catheter in the lumen, information which is not obtainable from the angiogram alone. Therefore, current research is examining whether an ultrasound image-based dosing algorithm can optimize therapeutic benefit[167,168].

In follow-up studies after brachytherapy and drug-eluting stents it is extremely important to analyze the worst lesion site as well as adjacent segments, because the bulk of the restenotic tissue may not localize at the worst pre-interventional lesion site and/or the treatment may have effects at the non-treated borders[167]. Important examples are arterial remodeling[168,169] and the 'candy wrapper' effect after brachytherapy[166].

7

Evolving clinical and research applications

Over the past few years, several new applications of IVUS have emerged, which have already enhanced our understanding of atherosclerotic plaque development. Two important areas are the focal assessment of plaque composition and stability and the assessment of overall plaque burden.

7.1 ASSESSMENT OF PLAQUE VULNERABILITY
(FIGURES 102–116, 138–161)

Rupture or superficial erosion of vulnerable coronary plaques with subsequent thrombosis represents the principal pathophysiology underlying most acute coronary syndromes[170–175]. Plaque vulnerability describes a temporary activated state of athero-sclerotic plaques, leading to a higher risk of plaque rupture and thrombosis[176–178]. Most vulnerable plaques stabilize either without rupture or after episodes of clinically inapparent rupture and subsequent fibrosis, and only in a few cases do rupture and thrombosis lead to vessel occlusion and acute coronary syndromes[179–181]. The patho-physiologic processes responsible for plaque destabilization are incompletely understood, but systemic, and in particular inflammatory, triggers play an important role[175,182]. The role of systemic triggers is supported by the recent observation that plaque destabilization in patients presenting with acute coronary syndromes is characterized by the diffuse development of multiple vulnerable lesions simultaneously (FIGURES 109, 110, 115, 116)[85,182–188].

The *in vivo* identification of vulnerable plaques before rupture would allow the development of systemic and local interventions directed at plaque stabilization. However, because vulnerable lesions are a temporary stage in plaque development, their temporal and spatial distribution in the entire coronary tree is highly dynamic and dependent on the clinical situation. The assessment of plaque vulnerability using IVUS therefore faces two challenges: the morphological characterization of *focal* vulnerable lesions but also the assessment of the *systemic* disease process[29,186].

7.1.1 Morphology of focal, severely stenotic culprit lesions in patients with stable and unstable presentation
(FIGURES 102–107)

Initial IVUS studies have compared plaque charac-teristics of focal, highly stenotic culprit lesions of patients presenting with stable and unstable coronary syndromes. Plaque echolucency, which correlates with increased lipid content of plaques, has been associated with unstable clinical present-ation (unstable angina and acute myocardial infarction) (FIGURE 102)[88–91]. Recent studies describe a consistent association between unstable clinical presentation and expansive (positive) arterial remodeling (FIGURES 103 AND 104)[64,65,92–96].

Our group compared pre-interventional IVUS images of patients with stable and unstable clinical presentation. The unstable group included 61 patients with unstable angina and 24 patients with recent or acute myocardial infarction. The stable group included 46 patients with stable angina. The direction of remodeling was consistently related to clinical presentation. Expansive (positive) remodel-ing was significantly more common in the unstable group (51.8% vs. 19.6%, $p = 0.001$), and constrictive (negative) remodeling was more common in the stable group (56.5% vs. 31.8%, $p = 0.001$). The remodeling ratio was significantly greater in the unstable group than in the stable group (1.06 ± 0.2 versus 0.94 ± 0.2, $p = 0.008$). Echolucent plaques were more frequent in the unstable than in the stable group (19% vs. 4 %, $p = 0.02$)[64].

Other studies reveal a consistent pattern. A comparative angioscopic and intracoronary ultrasound study found an association of angioscopic complex lesions with expansive enlargement and unstable presentation[92]. In histological studies, evidence of plaque inflammation is associated with larger plaque and EEM areas in femoral and coronary arteries[65,188,190,191]. These results suggest that expansive (positive) arterial remodeling is associated with lesions characterized by an increased risk of plaque rupture.

A group of enzymes, the matrix metalloproteinases (MMP), appears to play an important role in both positive remodeling and plaque instability[192,193]. This group of enzymes is central in the continuous production and degradation of matrix components[194–196]. Our group investigated the relation between MMP staining and direction of remodeling in human coronary lesions. We performed *in vivo* IVUS and subsequently used directional coronary atherectomy (DCA) to obtain histological specimens of the imaged lesion site in 35 patients[197]. MMP presence was associated with macrophages and smooth muscle cells. Intense cell-associated staining for MMP 3 was significantly more common in lesions with expansive arterial remodeling than in lesions with constrictive/intermediate remodeling (58% vs. 17%, $p = 0.04$). MMP 1, 2 and 9 were not different between lesions with expansive and constrictive/intermediate remodeling.

Histological studies have been performed in femoral and coronary arteries confirming the relation between inflammation, MMP and remodeling[198-202]. These results suggest that the degradation of extracellular matrix by MMP and other proteolytic enzymes may contribute to the expansion of the coronary vessel wall, which is characteristic of expansive (positive) remodeling. Conversely, the fibrotic changes associated with constrictive (negative) remodeling[203] may increase internal plaque resistance to rupture. Thus, a paradox may exist in which expansive (positive) remodeling protects against luminal narrowing, but increases the likelihood of a cascade of events leading to plaque

rupture[65]. The balance between inflammation and fibrosis may be an important determinant of plaque progression/regression and vulnerability[204].

7.1.2 The rationale for prospective studies of mildly stenotic lesions
(FIGURES 108–110)

Most current knowledge about the morphology of vulnerable plaques has been derived from plaques that had already ruptured. In these studies, vulnerable plaques are characterized by a necrotic core, separated from the lumen by a thin fibrous cap. It is conceivable that these paradigms about morphological changes of individual vulnerable plaques, based on autopsy studies of fatal coronary events, are not applicable to *in vivo* imaging of non-fatal cases[85]. The overwhelming evidence that most vulnerable lesions are not highly stenotic demonstrates that it is necessary to identify characteristics of vulnerability in mildly stenotic lesions before rupture. Only such prospective studies can determine if morphological characteristics including echolucency and the extent and direction of arterial remodeling can *predict* the risk of developing acute coronary syndromes.

Most of the above-mentioned imaging results have been derived from severely stenotic 'culprit lesions' examined at the time of coronary intervention (FIGURES 106 AND 107). However, it is well known that pre-existing severe stenosis does not predict the site of future events[205–211]. In fact, most acute coronary events are initiated from previously mildly stenotic lesion sites.

Results from IVUS studies examining mildly stenotic lesion are limited. Mildly stenotic lesions are commonly found in the coronary tree of asymptomatic persons[114,212]. It is unclear why certain lesions suddenly become destabilized and progress to rupture and thrombosis (FIGURES 108–110)[85,179–189].

A recent prospective IVUS study of early, angiographically mildly stenotic lesions described characteristic remodeling patterns of vulnerable plaques before rupture[96]. A total of 114 coronary sites without significant stenosis by angiography (< 50% diameter stenosis) were identified and examined with IVUS at baseline. During 2 years follow-up, 12 patients had an acute coronary event caused by a previously examined site. These 'vulnerable' sites were compared with lesions that did not cause acute events. At baseline, the vulnerable sites more frequently exhibited echolucent morphology and larger plaque areas with similar lumen areas, suggesting expansive (positive) remodeling.

Our group analyzed remodeling response in 251 mildly stenotic focal lesions (50% or less diameter stenosis by angiography) using IVUS[213]. At the lesion and proximal reference site, EEM area, lumen area, and plaque area were determined. The remodeling ratio (RR) was calculated by dividing the EEM area at the lesion by that at the proximal reference site. Expansive (positive) and constrictive (negative) remodeling were defined as RR of 1.05, and 0.95, respectively. We found expansive (positive) remodeling in 116 lesions (46%) and constrictive (negative) remodeling in 66 (26%). Plaque and lumen area were significantly larger in lesions with expansive (positive) than constrictive (negative) remodeling ($p = 0.04$ and 0.0019). These results demonstrate that expansive (positive) and constrictive (negative) remodeling does frequently occur in mildly stenotic lesions of native coronary artery disease. The clinical significance is incompletely understood.

7.1.3 IVUS and other imaging modalities

While IVUS and other invasive imaging modalities, including optical coherence tomography and thermography, are important tools in clinical research[27], non-invasive techniques will eventually be necessary to apply atherosclerosis imaging in a preventive setting. CT and MRI are currently areas of intense research, but it is important to emphasize that their resolution is significantly lower than IVUS[29–31,214,215] and it would therefore be unrealistic to expect clinical applications for the assessment of coronary plaque vulnerability in the near future.

7.2 ASSESSMENT OF DISEASE BURDEN/VOLUMETRIC ANALYSIS
(FIGURES 117–125)

While the characterization of focal atherosclerotic lesions is important for the assessment of plaque composition and stability, pathological studies show that coronary artery disease is a systemic process, with a multifocal distribution in the coronary tree[212]. IVUS studies confirm *in vivo* that plaque distribution is more diffuse than anticipated based on the angiographic appearance of focal stenosis (FIGURES 115, 116, 119, 120)[74,75,114]. The reason for the discrepancy between angiographic and tomographic

imaging methods is the process of outward expansion of the EEM area (expansive remodeling) in early stages of coronary artery disease, allowing plaque development without luminal compromise[55,56] (Chapter 5.1.2).

There are several approaches to examine the diffuse disease process. The comparison of sequential lesions in the same artery could improve the understanding of local and systemic factors influencing disease progression/regression. The overall assessment of plaque burden will allow the quantitative assessment of plaque progression and regression.

7.2.1 Sequential lesions
(FIGURES 115, 116, 177, 178)

It is unknown whether sequential lesions in the same coronary artery have similar characteristics in regard to morphology, remodeling and vulnerability. Similar characteristics would suggest the predominant effect of systemic triggers; different characteristics would attest to the prominent role of focal factors. We examined 1002 angiographically mildly diseased coronary arteries and could identify 44 arteries with pairs of clearly delineated sequential lesions[216]. For each lesion, we measured the lumen and external elastic membrane (EEM) areas, at both target lesion and normal proximal reference sites. Plaque area and percentage CSA area stenosis were calculated. The remodeling ratio (RR) and expansive (positive) and constrictive (negative) remodeling were defined as described above. We found that the frequencies of expansive (positive) and constrictive (negative) remodeling were similar at the proximal and distal lesions in the overall group. However, the correlation of the RR between proximal and distal lesions was weak ($R = 0.334$) and there was no relation of the remodeling categories between proximal and distal lesions (χ^2, $p = 0.3$). These preliminary results demonstrate that the remodeling response of sequential lesions in adjacent vessel segments is independent. The biological relevance of this finding is unclear, but suggests that local factors play an important role in modulating arterial remodeling.

7.2.2 Volumetric analysis (FIGURES 35,128,129)

In order to assess the overall disease process, it is necessary to analyze the spatial distribution of plaque burden and remodeling response along entire vessel segments[68,69,217,218]. For quantitative, volumetric assessment of plaque burden, consecutive plaque area measurements performed at known distances are integrated along a vessel segment (Chapter 4.8). The ability of IVUS to precisely quantify the extent of atherosclerotic plaque burden is currently examined in serial regression–progression trials, in which plaque burden is the primary end- point (FIGURES 35,128,129)[68,69] (Chapter 7.3).

The prognostic role of plaque burden is not completely understood. However, it is an attractive hypothesis that the effect of systemic triggers causes more instability when acting upon a larger plaque mass, therefore increasing the statistical chance of a clinical event. The assessment of plaque burden may, therefore, be an important component in the assessment of plaque vulnerability.

7.3 SERIAL EXAMINATION OF PROGRESSION–REGRESSION
(FIGURES 126–178)

7.3.1 Matching (FIGURES 126–161)

Serial IVUS examination of the same lesion site or vessel segment can provide important insights into the progression and regression of coronary artery disease. Serial studies require matching of the examined vessel site or segment to compared follow-up and baseline studies. Traditionally, individual images have been compared side by side, using angiographic and IVUS landmarks (side-branches, pericardium, and cardiac veins) to match sites (FIGURES 126 AND 127). The comparison of individual sites allows observation of temporal development of plaque morphology and size. Figures 130–161 show examples of individual matched lesion sites at baseline and follow-up demonstrating many of the morphologic criteria described in earlier chapters. The potential value but also the limitations of this approach are outlined in the accompanying figure text.

A more precise quantitative approach of matching is used in volumetric IVUS progression–regression trials. In these studies, motorized pullback sequences of entire coronary segments, selected between two fiduciary points, are matched and compared (FIGURES 128 AND 129) (Chapter 4.8). A target segment of a vessel is identified, the ultrasound catheter is placed distal to a fiduciary point such as a coronary branch, and a motorized pullback is performed. Using the fiduciary side-branch as the starting point, evenly spaced images (typically at 1 mm distance) are analyzed. Studies show that plaque plus medial volume calculated in this manner is highly reproducible and that serial studies can detect very small changes in atheroma volume[68,69,219]. These studies allow assessment of disease progression and regression.

7.3.2 Progression and regression
(FIGURES 162–178)

The detection and quantification of subclinical coronary atherosclerosis could allow serial monitoring during various therapeutic interventions[68,69]. In transplant vasculopathy, regression has occasionlly been observed[220], and volumetric studies showed decreased disease progression with novel immunosuppressive medications[124]. Other studies have demonstrated complex serial changes of plaque and EEM area after transplantation[221,222]. In native coronary artery disease using matched individual images, the progression of plaque area has been examined in a small study investigating the effect of 3-year treatment with pravastatin or diet in mildly diseased coronary arteries[223]. Follow-up plaque area increased by 41% in the control group but decreased by 7% in the treatment group. In a similar study, the effect of low density lipoprotein (LDL) apharesis on plaque regression was examined. Plaque area decreased in the LDL apharesis groups (from 8.45 ± 4.22 mm^2 to 7.76 ± 4.34 mm^2) over a 1-year follow-up period, but increased in the control group (from 7.19 ± 2.88 mm^2 to 8.08 ± 3.14 mm^2)[224]. In a serial, volumetric IVUS analysis, Schartl and colleagues described plaque volume and plaque morphology in a serial IVUS study during lipid-lowering treatment[219]. A total of 131 patients were randomized to treatment with atorvastatin or 'usual care', which could include statin therapy. After 12 months, mean LDL-cholesterol was reduced from 155 to 86 mg/dl in the atorvastatin group and from 166 to 140 mg/dl in the 'usual care' group. Mean absolute plaque volume showed a statistically insignificant smaller increase in the atorvastatin group compared with the 'usual care' group (1.2 ± 30 versus 49.6 ± 28.1 mm^3, $p = 0.19$). Echogenicity increased to a larger extent in the atorvastatin group than in the 'usual care' group. Several other large IVUS regression–progression studies are currently underway[68,69].

These include the Reversal of Atherosclerosis with Lipitor (REVERSAL) trial (657 patients), which is comparing two lipid-lowering regimens (expected completion, 2003), and the Norvasc for Regression of Manifest Atherosclerotic Lesions (NORMALISE) trial (450 patients), which is comparing amlodipine, enalapril, and placebo (expected completion, 2003). In both studies, IVUS measurements of plaque burden represent the primary end-point. Such studies avoid the inherent limitations of angiographic regression trials and have the potential to define a new standard for the evaluation of drug therapy to limit the progression of atherosclerosis. Figures 162–178 show examples of progression and regression in individually matched lesions. Figures 180–190 show case studies of progression and regression.

Prospective evidence that coronary plaque burden correlates with future clinical events is not available. However, studies using carotid ultrasound demonstrate that intimal media thickness is correlated with clinical events[225].

8

Conclusion

Our understanding of the pathophysiology of coronary artery disease and, in particular, acute coronary syndromes has significantly evolved over the last decade[172–178]. In addition to understanding the mechanical and hemodynamic significance of severe stenosis, supported by angiography and other *in vivo* diagnostic tools, we now understand the cellular, molecular and genetic biology of atherosclerotic plaques before rupture. This expanding information has also influenced the approach to imaging of coronary atherosclerosis with invasive and non-invasive modalities[29–31,85,226-228] (FIGURE 179). The precise evaluation of individual severely stenotic lesions remains important in order to define the need and approach of revascularization. On the other hand, identification of lesion vulnerability and quantification of plaque burden are emerging as tools of risk assessment[189].

IVUS is an established clinical tool used in a wide variety of settings, ranging from more traditional indications related to percutaneous coronary interventions to emerging applications in atherosclerosis imaging. In this Manual, we have described this spectrum of IVUS applications and their importance in clinical applications.

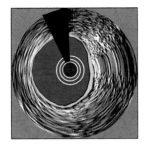

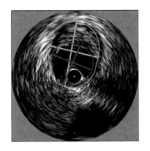

Section 2

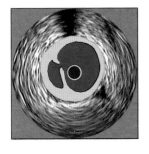

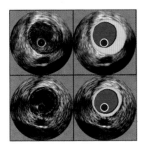

The Atlas of
Coronary Intravascular
Ultrasound Imaging

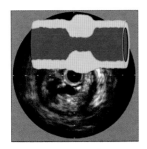

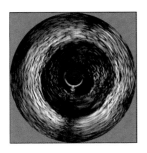

Basics of IVUS: introduction

Intravascular ultrasound (IVUS) is a tomographic imaging modality performed during coronary angiography. IVUS imaging allows the simultaneous assessment of lumen, vessel wall, and atherosclerotic plaque. Therefore, IVUS is complementary to selective coronary angiography, which is limited to a longitudinal silhouette of the lumen.

The experience with IVUS imaging has provided important insights into the anatomy of atherosclerotic lesion development and can guide patient management in different clinical situations. Clinical, interventional indications to perform IVUS are ambiguous angiographic findings and the guidance of percutaneous coronary intervention (PCI). In addition, IVUS has been established as the method of choice for the detection and serial observation of transplant vasculopathy and, more recently, serial observation of plaque burden in atherosclerosis regression–progression trials.

This Atlas illustrates the rationale, technique, and interpretation of IVUS imaging in diagnostic and therapeutic applications.

CHAPTER 1, REFERENCES 1–10

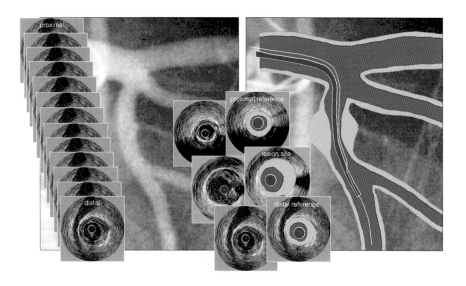

Figure 1   Principle of IVUS examination
Intravascular ultrasound (IVUS) is an invasive tomographic imaging modality. During cardiac catheterization, a coronary IVUS catheter is advanced over a guidewire beyond the target lesion. The pullback through the lesion or segment of interest results in a series of cross-sectional images.

Using a typical pullback speed of 0.5 mm/s and a frame-rate of 30 images/s, 60 images will be available from a pullback through a 1-mm segment. Typically, a subsample of these images is analyzed depending on the clinical indication.

The six IVUS cross-sections on the right demonstrate the identification of the worst lesion site and adjacent proximal and distal reference sites. This approach is often used for the guidance of interventional procedures.

The multiple IVUS images on the left demonstrate the approach taken for volumetric IVUS examinations. Several images are obtained at constant intervals, allowing three-dimensional reconstruction and volumetric analysis.

CHAPTER 1.1, REFERENCES 1, 9, 10

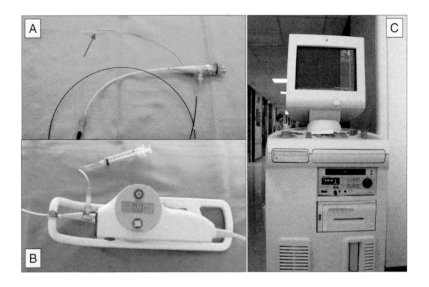

Figure 2   IVUS equipment
The equipment required to perform intracoronary ultrasound consists of three major components: a catheter (A) incorporating a miniaturized ultrasound transducer (red arrow), a pullback device (B), and the IVUS console (C).

The imaging console includes the hard- and software to convert the IVUS signal to the image, the monitor and recording devices. Imaging studies are usually recorded on videotape, but newer systems permit digital recording and permanent archiving on CD-ROM.

CHAPTER 1.2, REFERENCES 9, 10

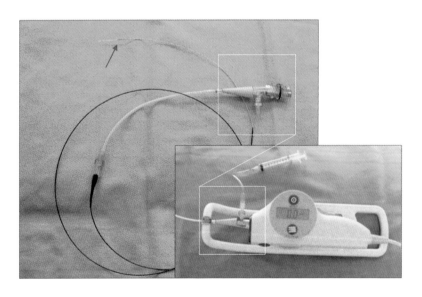

Figure 3   IVUS equipment: catheter and motorized pullback sled
Current catheters range in size from 2.6 to 3.5 French (0.87–1.17 mm) and can be placed through a 6-French guiding catheter. Mechanical and electronic catheter designs are used. Mechanical probes use a drive cable to rotate a single ultrasound transducer at 1800 rpm. In contrast, electronic systems consist of multiple transducer elements (up to 64) in an annular array, which are activated sequentially to generate the image.

The pullback is performed either manually or using a motorized pullback device. Motorized pullback devices withdraw the catheter at a constant speed of 0.5–1.0 mm/s.

CHAPTERS 1.2 AND 1.3.3, REFERENCES 9, 10

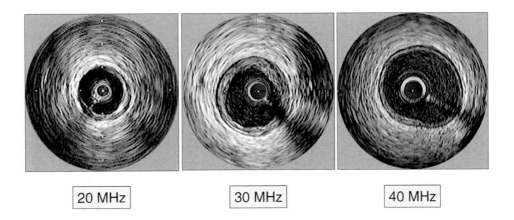

20 MHz   30 MHz   40 MHz

Figure 4   IVUS equipment: catheter frequency and resolution
The ultrasound frequencies used in current catheter systems are centered at 20–50 MHz. At 30 MHz, axial resolution is 150 μm and lateral resolution averages 250 μm.

These three images show the difference in image quality between catheters with different imaging frequency. While the higher resolution of 40 MHz catheters allows better detail differentiation of the vessel wall, the signal speckle from the intraluminal blood is more prominent. This artifact can blur the border between the lumen and the intima.

CHAPTER 1.2.1, REFERENCES 9, 10

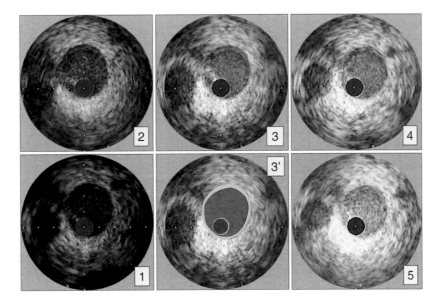

Figure 5   System settings: gain
Systems setting are very important in order to avoid misinterpretation of IVUS findings. Gain refers to amplification of the returned signal. Increasing the overall gain can compensate for a low sensitivity catheter, but at the expense of creating images with increased noise and decreased gray-scale information.

In this figure, the same image is shown while the gain is gradually increased (panels 1–5). Panel 3' illustrates the findings from panel 3.

CHAPTER 1.3.2, REFERENCES 9, 10

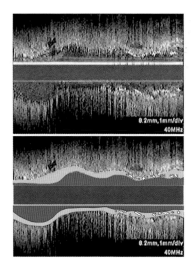 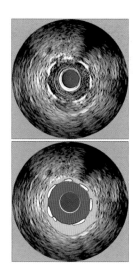

Figure 6   IVUS display
The standard display of IVUS systems consists of individual cross-sectional images reviewed individually and as a video sequence (right panels).

Motorized transducer pullback and digital storage of cross-sectional images are necessary for longitudinal image reconstruction (L-mode; left panels). However, there are major limitations to the L-mode display. The changes of vessel size during the cardiac cycle result in a characteristic artifact described as the 'saw-tooth' appearance. ECG-triggered image acquisition of image frames in the same cardiac phase may eliminate this artifact.

Length measurements can be performed using the L-mode display. However, missing information about the three-dimensional vessel curvature in the L-mode is a limitation of these measurements.

CHAPTERS 1.3.4 AND 4.7, REFERENCES 14–19

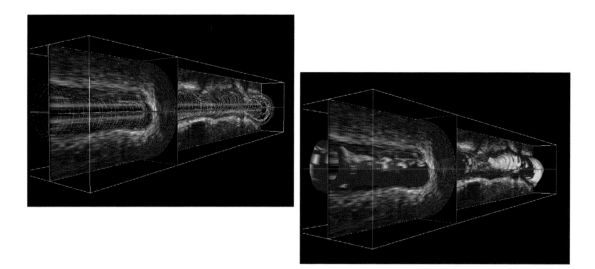

Figure 7   Three-dimensional display
Scrolling through adjacent cross-sectional images of a pullback sequence allows the experienced operator to obtain a three-dimensional impression of the vessel segment.

Automated, three-dimensional reconstruction of IVUS involves the use of advanced computer rendering techniques to display a shaded or wire-frame image of the vessel. However, true three-dimensional techniques require registration of the catheter path during the pullback. These methods are not yet included in current clinical systems but are an exciting area of research.

CHAPTER 1.3.4, REFERENCES 14–19

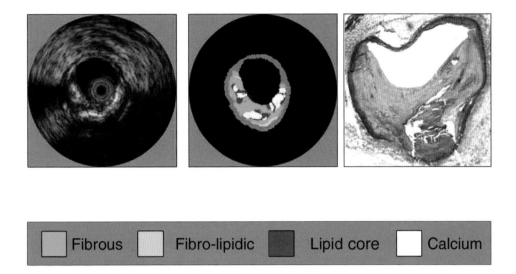

Figure 8   Radiofrequency analysis

The raw IVUS signal is converted for conventional image presentation on the standard display. Additional analysis of the reflected ultrasound signal, analyzing several characteristics of the digitized ultrasound signal with integrated radiofrequency analysis, backscatter analysis, and elastography, allows advanced tissue characterization and more objective and reproducible methods of categorizing wall morphology and plaque components. However, the clinical value of these advanced image analysis modalities is not completely defined.

CHAPTER 1.3.5, REFERENCES 20–27

Arterial anatomy

The following figures demonstrate how the structures of the arterial wall are reflected in the IVUS image.

CHAPTER 2, REFERENCES 1–10, 32–37

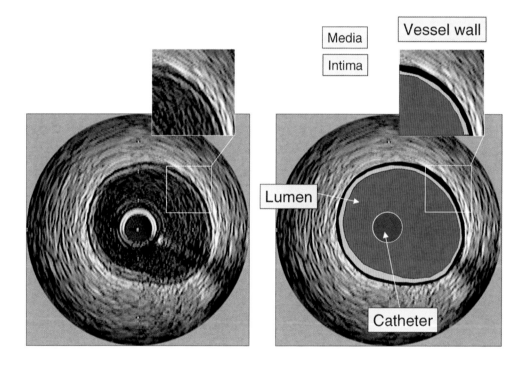

Figure 9   Normal lumen and arterial wall
IVUS allows a detailed view of the arterial wall with a spatial resolution of about 150–250 μm. In the IVUS image, the catheter is centered in the vessel, surrounded by the lumen, vessel wall and adjacent structures.

The fine 'speckle' caused by reflections of the ultrasound at flowing erythrocytes, differentiates lumen and vessel wall. In high-quality images, the vessel wall shows three layers: the echodense intima, the echolucent media and the more echodense adventitia. However, the normal media often cannot be differentiated.

CHAPTER 2, REFERENCES 9, 10, 32–36

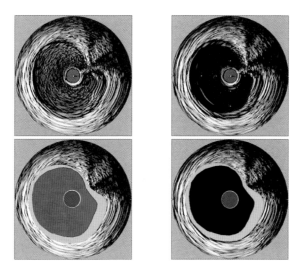

Figure 10   Lumen

At frequencies > 20 MHz, flowing blood exhibits a characteristic pattern of echogenicity, observed as finely textured echoes moving in a swirling pattern in video sequences. This blood 'speckle' assists in differentiating between the lumen and vessel wall.

Flushing of the vessel with saline or contrast during IVUS imaging can help to differentiate the lumen and vessel wall by providing a uniform signal during the injection, as shown in the image on the right (saline flush).

CHAPTER 2.1, REFERENCES 9, 10

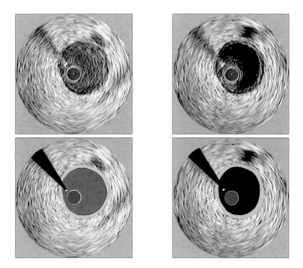

Figure 11   Lumen, saline flush

Blood speckle is more prominent at higher imaging frequencies, and may interfere with delineation of the blood–tissue interface. The effect of flushing of the vessel with saline is more obvious in these situations, as shown in the images on the right.

CHAPTER 2.1, REFERENCES 9, 10

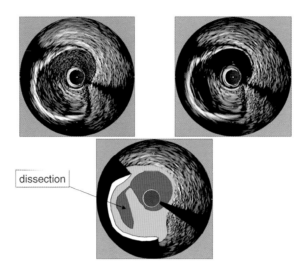

Figure 12   Dissection plane, saline flush

Flushing of the artery with saline or contrast during IVUS imaging can also help to differentiate the communication between a dissection plane and the lumen and demonstrate blood flow in a double lumen, as shown here.

CHAPTER 2.1, REFERENCES 9, 10

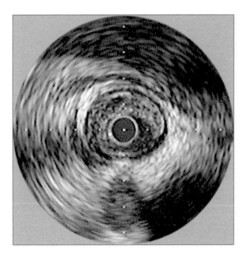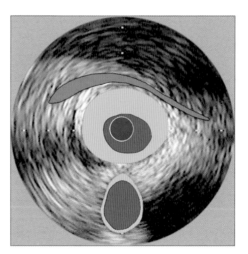

Figure 13   Adjacent structures

Depending on the size of the artery, adjacent structures including arterial side-branches, cardiac veins, and the pericardium can be differentiated.

   These structures are frequently used as landmarks for the matching in serial studies (see Chapter 7.3.1). In this figure, the pericardial space is shown in blue and an arterial side-branch is seen at the 6 o'clock position.

CHAPTER 2.3, REFERENCES 9, 10, 37

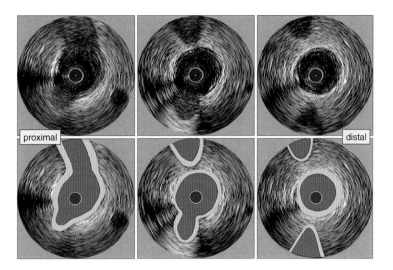

Figure 14   Arterial side-branches
During the transducer pullback through the vessel, arterial side-branches characteristically appear at the periphery of the image and then join the imaged vessel.

 Sequential images of a pullback sequence are shown. Two arterial side-branches (diagonal and septal branch) are seen joining the left anterior descending artery.

CHAPTER 2.3, REFERENCES 9, 10, 37

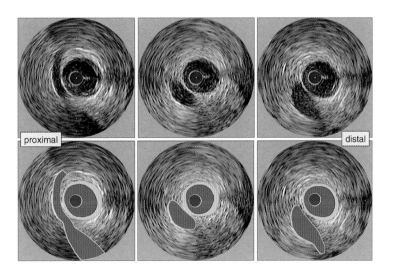

Figure 15   Cardiac veins (1)
In contrast to arterial side-branches, cardiac veins run parallel to the artery or cross the artery, but characteristically do not join the imaged vessel.

 Sequential images of a pullback sequence are shown. A vein crosses the vessel at the 7 o'clock position.

CHAPTER 2.3, REFERENCES 9, 10, 37

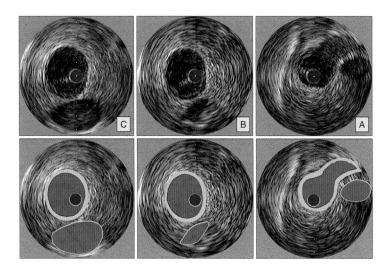

Figure 16   Cardiac veins (2)

Cardiac veins can be differentiated from arterial side-branches by the systolic collapse (panel C (diastole) and B (systole)) and by the fact that veins cross but do not join the artery (panel A, showing an arterial side-branch joining the vessel, while the vein crosses).

The identification of cardiac veins is important in the recently described percutaneous *in situ* coronary artery bypass (PICAB) procedure. In this percutaneous coronary revascularization technique, a conduit is created between a proximal coronary vessel and a coronary vein.

CHAPTER 2.3, REFERENCES 9, 10, 37, 38

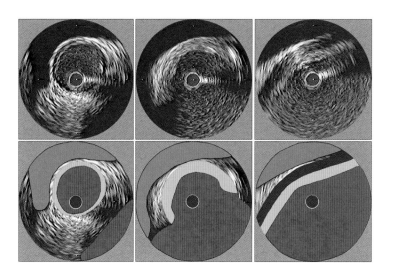

Figure 17   Bifurcation: left main aorta–ostium

The proximal segment of a side-branch, joining the imaged vessel, can often be evaluated during the IVUS pullback. However, because of the eccentric position of the catheter, these images are difficult to interpret.

Transducer obliquity and eccentric position can result in an overestimation of measured dimensions and a reduction in image quality, as shown here for the wall of the aorta at the aorto–ostial bifurcation. The ultrasound beam strikes the vessel wall in a shallow angle, producing the thickened wall with different echogenicity.

CHAPTERS 2.4 AND 3.6, REFERENCES 9, 10, 48

Image artifacts

Imaging artifacts are common and are important to understand for the proper interpretation of images. The most common artifacts are explained in the following images.

CHAPTER 3, REFERENCES 45–50

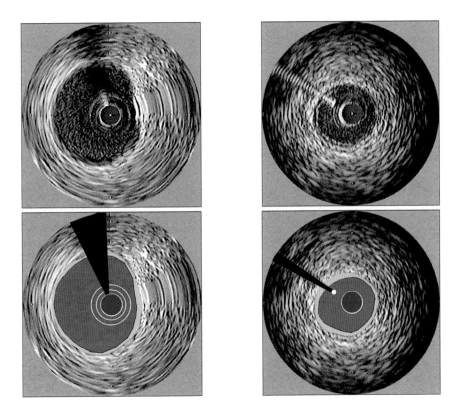

Figure 18   Guide-wire artifact
Using monorail catheter technology, the guide-wire lies outside of the transducer and causes a typical artifact, which is characterized by a narrow-angled shadow. Depending on the settings and operating frequency, these artifacts can be echolucent (left panels) or echodense (right panels).

CHAPTER 3.1, REFERENCES 9, 10, 45

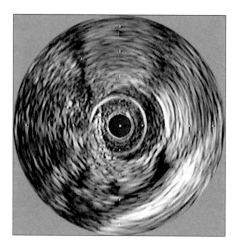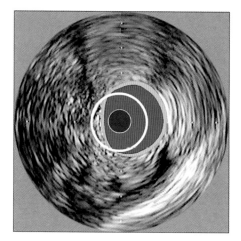

Figure 19   Ring-down artifact

Ring-down artifacts are usually observed as bright halos of variable thickness surrounding the catheter.

They are caused by acoustic oscillations in the transducer, which result in high-amplitude ultrasound signals that obscure the area immediately adjacent to the catheter.

Ring-down artifacts create a zone of diagnostic uncertainty adjacent to the transducer surface.

CHAPTER 3.2, REFERENCES 9, 10, 45

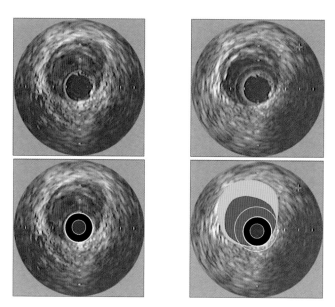

Figure 20   Imaging artifacts: digital subtraction (1)

Electronic transducer systems allow image optimization performed at the beginning of the pullback. Ring-down is partially reduced by digital subtraction of a reference mask. If it is incorrectly performed, digital subtraction has the potential to remove relevant tissue reflections or introduce false borders.

The above images were obtained with an electronic IVUS/Doppler catheter combination. Blood flow is shown in red on the left-hand images and allows the visualization of the digital subtraction effect. The signal-free space surrounding the catheter is an artifact introduced by sub-optimal digital subtraction.

CHAPTER 3.2, REFERENCES 9, 10, 45

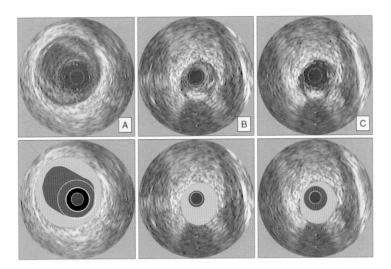

Figure 21   Imaging artifacts: digital subtraction (2)
This figure demonstrates the effect of incorrect digital subtraction.
In these images, different levels of digital subtraction cause an apparent change in luminal size. Images of the proximal reference are shown in panel A, and images of the lesion in panels B and C. The lesion appears tighter in panel B than in panel C, which are taken at exactly the same site during the process of digital subtractions. The apparently larger lumen in panel C is caused by artificial signal drop-out around the catheter.

CHAPTER 3.2, REFERENCES 9, 10, 45

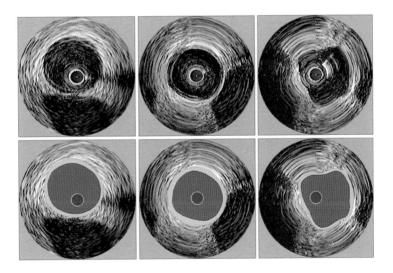

Figure 22   Imaging artifacts: non-uniform rotational distortion
An important artifact, 'non-uniform rotational distortion'(NURD), arises from uneven drag on the drive cable of mechanical catheters, resulting in cyclical oscillations in rotational transducer speed, observed as visible distortion of the image.
NURD can occur for a number of reasons, including the presence of acute bends in the artery, tortuous guiding catheter shapes, kinking of the imaging sheath, or small lumen of the guiding catheter. A frequent, reversible cause is excessive tightening of the hemostatic valve.

CHAPTER 3.3, REFERENCES 9, 10, 45

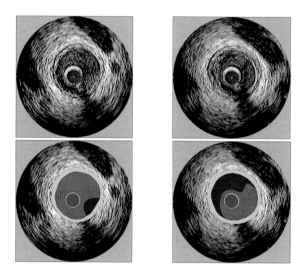

Figure 23   Image artifact: slow flow versus thrombus
The intensity of the blood speckle increases exponentially as blood flow velocity decreases. Therefore, flow stagnation can limit the ability to differentiate lumen from echolucent tissue, including soft plaque, neointima, and thrombus. This artifact is often encountered when the catheter is advanced across a tight stenosis.
In this figure, the brown-shaded areas were interpreted as an intracoronary thrombus.

CHAPTER 3.4, REFERENCES 9, 10, 82

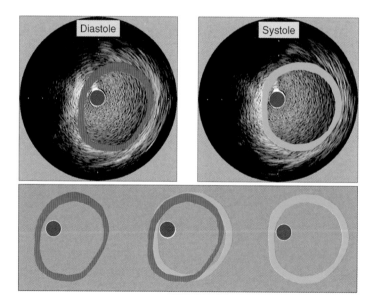

Figure 24   Image artifacts: coronary pulsation
The changes of pressure and flow in the coronary circulation lead to characteristic changes of arterial size and shape during the cardiac cycle. Systolic and diastolic frames are shown in the upper part of this figure. The difference in size and shape of the vessel is illustrated in the graphics below. In normal arteries, the diameter is maximal in systole, although flow is maximal in diastole, when resistance to flow in the small intramyocardial vessels is minimal.

CHAPTER 3.5, REFERENCES 46, 47

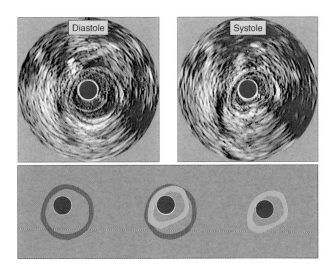

Figure 25   Image artifacts: muscle bridge
The cyclic pattern of artery size is reversed at the site of muscle bridges. Here, the artery size reaches a minimum during systole, caused by the contraction of the muscle surrounding the vessel.

CHAPTER 3.5, REFERENCES 9, 10, 37

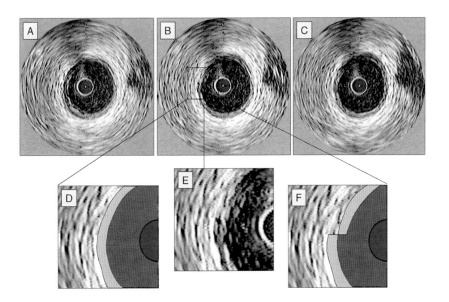

Figure 26   Imaging artifacts: partial image reconstruction
The IVUS image is reconstructed at 30 frames per second. Occasionally, part of an image results from two subsequent frames. This can introduce false borders, as shown in this example.

In this figure, three consecutive image frames (A, B, C) are shown. Frame B shows the effect of partial image reconstruction with the introduction of a characteristic step in the contour of the intima at the 9 o'clock position. This is illustrated in the illustrations (D, E, F).

The figure demonstrates that careful analysis of IVUS images always includes a review of adjacent images in order to recognize such artifacts.

CHAPTER 3.5, REFERENCES 9, 10

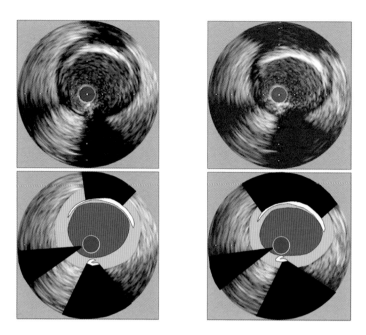

Figure 27 Imaging artifacts: calcium shadow

Calcium is an important part of atherosclerotic plaques and IVUS has a high sensitivity in its detection. However, almost all IVUS energy is reflected by calcium, causing a characteristic signal drop-out or multiple reflections of concentric arcs behind the calcified tissue. Therefore, the vessel wall behind calcified plaques cannot reliably be seen.

Calcium deposits are described qualitatively according to their location and distribution as superficial or deep. In addition, the arc of calcium can be measured in degrees.

CHAPTERS 3.7 AND 4.4, REFERENCES 9, 10, 49, 50

IVUS measurements

The following figures demonstrate standard measurements performed in individual IVUS images.

For IVUS measurement, manual or automated planimetry of the lumen–intima border and external elastic membrane border (EEM) is performed and distance and area measurements are derived.

In recent position papers from the AHA/ACC and ESC, these measurements have been reviewed and standardized.

CHAPTER 4, REFERENCES 9, 10

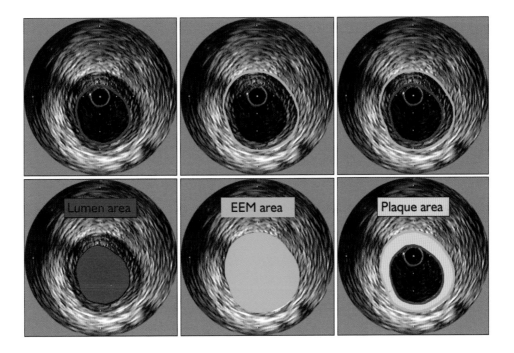

Figure 28   Area measurements, planimetry
The strong signal originating at the lumen–intima and external elastic membrane (EEM) border allow manual or automated planimetry of the lumen and EEM. Area measurements are calculated as follows:

Lumen CSA: the area bounded by the luminal border

EEM CSA: the area bounded by the adventitial border

Atheroma CSA: the EEM CSA minus the lumen CSA

CHAPTER 4, REFERENCES 9, 10

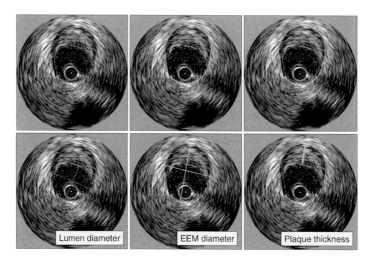

Figure 29   Circumference and diameter measurements

Once the lumen border and external elastic membrane (EEM) border have been delineated by planimetry, the following measurements are obtained.

Minimum and maximum lumen diameters: the shortest and longest diameters through the center point of the lumen

Minimum and maximum EEM diameters: the shortest and longest diameters through the center point of the EEM

Minimal and maximal plaque thicknesses are directly measured as the minimal and maximal distances between the lumen and EEM tracings.

CHAPTER 4, REFERENCES 9, 10

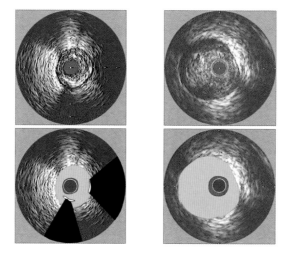

Figure 30   Plaque (atheroma) measurements

Atheroma measurements are derived by subtracting the lumen area from the EEM area.

Atheroma CSA: the EEM CSA minus the lumen CSA (FIGURE 28)

Maximum and minimum atheroma thicknesses: the largest or shortest distance from the intimal leading edge to the EEM along any line passing through the center of the lumen (FIGURE 29).

Atheroma burden: atheroma CSA divided by EEM CSA as a percentage. The atheroma burden represents the area within the EEM occupied by atheroma regardless of the luminal stenosis.

It should be realized that the atheroma burden, which is the percentage of the EEM area occupied by atheroma, is not equivalent to angiographic percentage stenosis, which represents an expression of luminal narrowing at the lesion relative to a reference segment.

In this figure, two highly stenotic lesion sites are shown. Importantly, the size of the plaque and the atheroma burden of the lesion in the right panels is significantly larger, despite the similar lumen dimensions (compare Figure 36).

CHAPTER 4.3, REFERENCES 9, 10

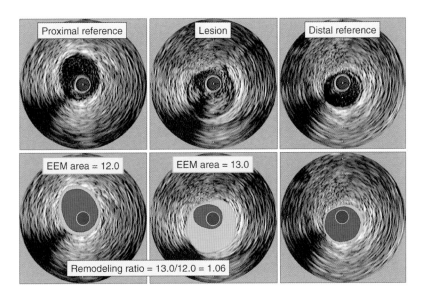

Figure 31 Remodeling measurements

Arterial remodeling refers to the changes in EEM area that occur during the development of atherosclerotic lesions.

The comparison of the EEM area at the lesion site with the EEM area at the proximal or distal reference site defines the remodeling response. A number of dichotomous definitions of remodeling have been proposed.

In this figure, the commonly used definition based on the comparison between the proximal reference and lesion site is shown. The remodeling ratio (RR) is calculated as:

RR = EEM lesion/EEM proximal reference

Expansive (positive), intermediate and constrictive (negative) remodeling are defined as RR > 1.05, 0.95–1.05, and < 0.95, respectively.

CHAPTER 4.5, REFERENCES 9, 10, 55–65

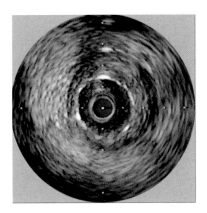 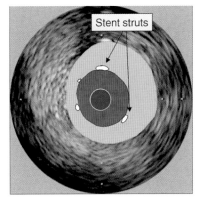

Figure 32   Coronary stent measurements

The stent adds an additional border to the IVUS image. The following measurements are commonly reported:

Stent CSA: the area bounded by the stent struts.

Maximum and minimum stent diameters: the longest and shortest diameters through the center of mass of the stent.

Stent symmetry: 100 x [(maximum stent diameter - minimum stent diameter) divided by maximum stent diameter].

Stent expansion: the minimum stent CSA compared with a reference area, which can be the proximal, distal, largest, or average reference area.

Strut apposition refers to the proximity of stent struts to the arterial wall. Good apposition is defined as sufficiently close contact to preclude blood flow between any strut and the underlying wall.

CHAPTER 4.6, REFERENCES 9, 10, 66, 67

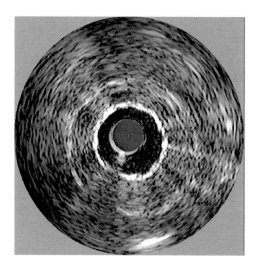 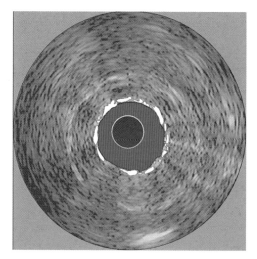

Figure 33   Covered stent

In this figure a stent covered with a plastic foil is shown. These stents have recently been introduced and are occasionally used for the treatment of vessel dissections. The foil causes a hazy shadow behind the stent.

CHAPTER 4.6, REFERENCES 9, 10

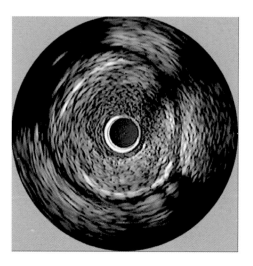 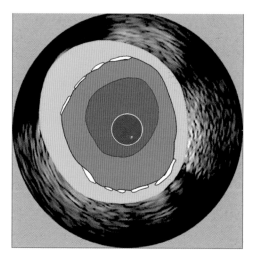

Figure 34   In-stent restenosis measurements

The neointimal tissue proliferation of in-stent restenosis is demonstrated in this figure by the orange color in the right image and is located inside the stent struts. Measurements of maximal and minimal thicknesses and areas of this tissue can be performed.

CHAPTER 4.6, REFERENCES 9, 10

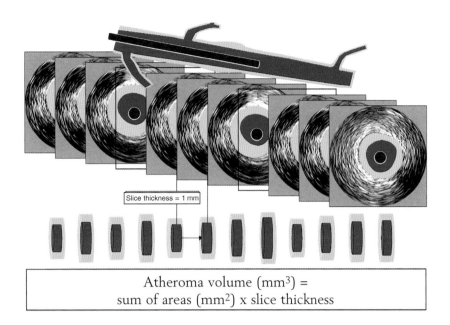

Slice thickness = 1 mm

Atheroma volume (mm³) =
sum of areas (mm²) x slice thickness

Figure 35   Quantitative volumetric IVUS analysis
For volumetric analysis of plaque burden, a segment of interest is selected between two characteristic fiduciary points (start- and end-point). Starting at the distal fiduciary location, evenly spaced single frames are selected from the digitized pullback sequence at 0.5–1.0-mm intervals. For each of the selected frames, the lumen and EEM cross-sectional areas are measured. The Simpson equation is applied to calculate plaque volume by multiplying plaque area and distance between adjacent images. An alternative approach is the ECG-gated/triggered selection of frames in a pre-defined relation to the cardiac cycle.

CHAPTERS 4.8 AND 7.2, REFERENCES 9, 10, 19, 68, 69, 219, 223, 224

Plaque (atheroma) morphology

Atheroma morphology describes characteristics of focal lesion sites.

Geometric characteristics are the relation between plaque size and severity of stenosis (mildly stenotic versus highly stenotic lesion), the longitudinal extent of the lesion (diffuse versus focal), the circumferential extent of the stenosis (eccentric versus concentric), and the extent and direction of remodeling.

Lesion echogenecity reflects underlying tissue composition. Typically, echolucent ('soft'), and echodense ('fibrous' and 'calcified') plaques are differentiated.

CHAPTER 5, REFERENCES 9, 10, 33–36

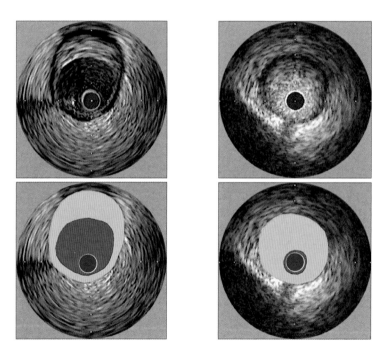

Figure 36   Geometry: lesion severity
A direct comparison between IVUS and angiography demonstrates that the extent and severity of disease by angiography and ultrasound are frequently discrepant. IVUS studies demonstrate that the size of the atheroma is not closely related to the size of the lumen. This phenomenon is a consequence of two major factors, the diffuse nature of atherosclerosis affecting the angiographically 'normal reference site' and adaptive enlargement of the EEM area (expansive or positive remodeling), which maintains lumen size despite plaque progression.

The complex relationship between plaque and lumen size is exemplified in this figure, which shows two lesions with similar plaque area. In the left-hand panels, the plaque is accommodated by expansion of the vessel size and has not led to luminal stenosis. In contrast, plaque accumulation has caused significant stenosis at the site of the lesion shown in the right-hand panels (compare to Figure 30).

CHAPTER 5.1.1, REFERENCES 55, 74, 75

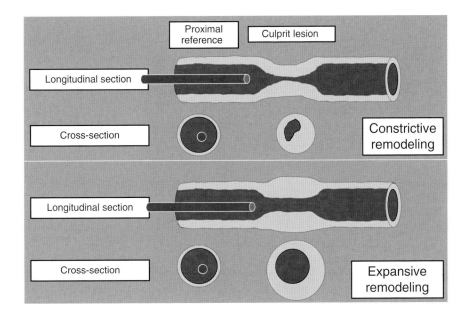

Figure 37   Geometry: arterial remodeling

The relation between plaque and lumen size is complex because of changes in vessel size (arterial remodeling) during lesion development. Arterial remodeling was initially described in necropsy specimens by Glagov and colleagues, who reported an expansion of the EEM area at atherosclerotic lesion sites (expansive or positive remodeling).

IVUS studies have subsequently confirmed these findings but also demonstrated the opposite process: constrictive or negative remodeling describes the shrinkage of the EEM area at diseased sites, contributing to luminal stenosis.

CHAPTER 5.1.2, REFERENCES 55–65

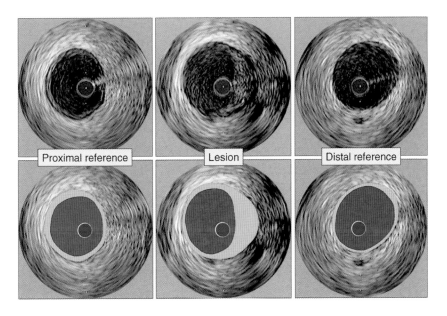

Figure 38   Expansive remodeling and early plaque accumulation

In a study examining postmortem human coronary arteries, Glagov and colleagues described a positive correlation between EEM and atheroma area for lesions with a stenosis < 40%. The authors hypothesized that this phenomenon represented a compensatory mechanism to preserve lumen size in early atherosclerotic lesions.

This image shows a mildly stenotic lesion with expansive remodeling, maintaining lumen size at the lesion site.

CHAPTER 5.1.2, REFERENCES 55, 56

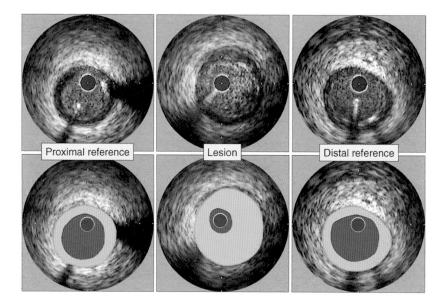

Figure 39 Expansive arterial remodeling
IVUS allows *in vivo* assessment of remodeling. Initial IVUS studies demonstrated expansive (positive) remodeling in severely stenotic culprit lesions. An example is shown in this figure. At the lesion site (middle panels), plaque accumulation is associated with an expansion of vessel size. The EEM area is larger at the lesion site than at the adjacent proximal reference site.

CHAPTER 5.1.2, REFERENCES 55–58

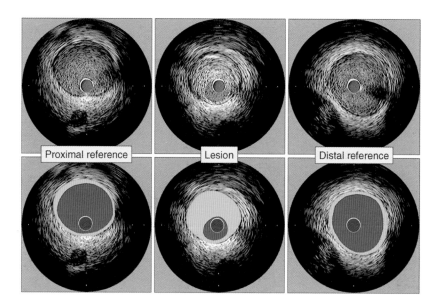

Figure 40 Constrictive arterial remodeling
Subsequent IVUS studies demonstrated shrinkage of the EEM area at the lesion site. This process is called constrictive or negative remodeling.

Constrictive remodeling was first described after percutaneous coronary intervention, but can also be observed in *de novo* lesions, contributing to luminal stenosis.

In this figure, a severely stenotic lesion with constrictive remodeling is shown. In contrast to the previous figure, the EEM area is smaller at the lesion site than at the adjacent reference site.

CHAPTER 5.1.2, REFERENCES 56, 59–63

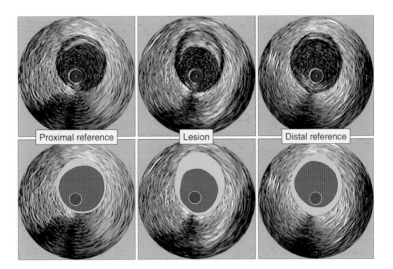

Figure 41 Remodeling and lesion stability

Several IVUS studies have examined the relationship between remodeling and clinical presentation in patients with coronary artery disease. In hemodynamically significant lesions, expansive remodeling is significantly more frequent in patients with unstable clinical presentation.

In a prospective study, expansive remodeling of mildly stenotic lesions at baseline was associated with an increased risk of acute coronary events during follow-up. Based on these results, it has been hypothesized that expansive arterial remodeling is related to vulnerability of mildly stenotic lesions (see Chapter 7.1).

This figure shows a mildly stenotic lesion with positive remodeling at the lesion site.

CHAPTER 5.1.2, REFERENCES 64, 65, 92–96, 188–191

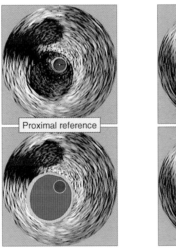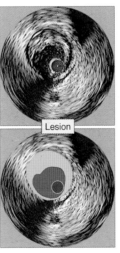

Figure 42 Constrictive remodeling: lesion stability

In contrast to Figure 41, this image shows a mildly stenotic lesion with negative remodeling. It has been suggested that the fibrotic changes associated with plaque healing/stabilization may cause negative remodeling.

CHAPTER 5.1.2, REFERENCES 64, 65, 92–96, 188–192

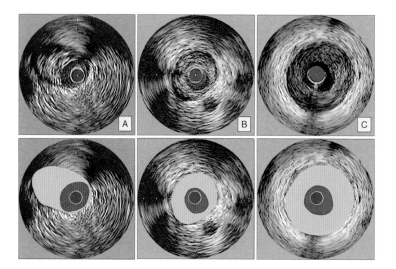

Figure 43   Geometry: eccentricity

The circumferential distribution of the atheroma is described by its eccentricity (see Chapter 4.3). Panel A shows an eccentric plaque and panel C a concentric plaque. Most lesions fall in between these two (panel B).

Early lesions and lesions at vessel bifurcations are characterized by eccentric distribution, suggesting a relation between local flow hemodynamics and lesion development.

CHAPTER 5.1.3, REFERENCES 39–44

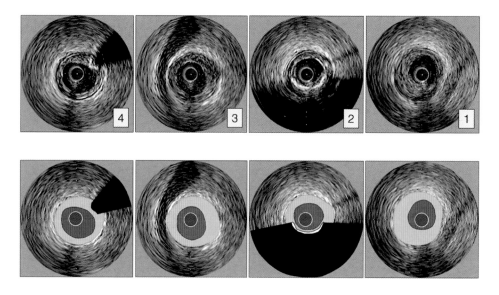

Figure 44   Geometry: diffuse disease

The strength of coronary angiography is the precise description of focal, severe luminal stenoses. However, it is well known that the atherosclerotic disease process is more diffuse, frequently reflected in angiographic 'mild luminal irregularities'. IVUS imaging has confirmed the diffuse character of coronary artery disease. It is difficult to describe the longitudinal extent of disease burden and there are currently no clear guidelines. An emerging approach is the description of plaque volumes in entire vessel segments (see Chapters 4.8 and 7.2).

These images show adjacent slices in a coronary segment with moderate diffuse plaque burden. Note that plaque is found in each of the four adjacent image slices but that morphology varies from echolucent (panel 3) to 'calcified' (panel 2).

CHAPTER 5.1.4, REFERENCES 9, 10, 74, 75

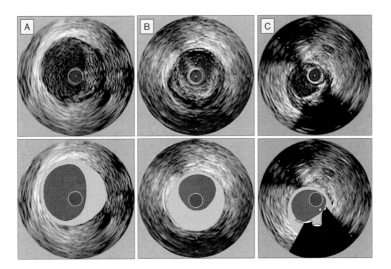

Figure 45 Plaque echogenicity

Ultrasound provides information about the morphology of atherosclerotic plaques *in vivo*. Lipid-rich lesions generate low-intensity, hypoechoic echoes (panel A). Fibrous tissues are relatively echogenic (panel B). Calcified plaques cause a characteristic acoustic shadowing (panel C).

Standard image interpretation relies on simple visual inspection of acoustic reflections to determine plaque composition. However, the texture of different tissue components may exhibit comparable acoustic properties and therefore appear quite similar by IVUS.

More objective and automated classification of atheromatous lesions is possible with advanced ultrasound data analysis. Radiofrequency analysis and elastography have been validated in *ex vivo* studies against histology and are emerging for clinical application (see Chapter 1.3.5).

CHAPTER 5.2, REFERENCES 9, 10, 20–27, 32-36, 76–78

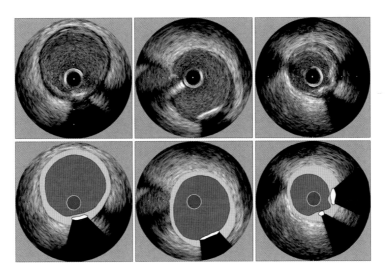

Figure 46 Calcified plaques

IVUS imaging has high sensitivity for the detection of coronary calcification. The significance of coronary calcifications is complex and the relation to plaque stability are unclear. Large calcifications may be associated with lesion stability. In contrast, microcalcifications, which are not well reflected in IVUS images, are frequently found in lipid-rich necrotic core areas of unstable plaques.

In this figure, several adjacent image slices of a calcified but mildly stenotic plaque are shown.

CHAPTER 5.2.3, REFERENCES 22, 49, 50, 80, 81

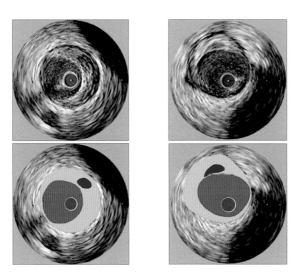

Figure 47   Mixed plaques, necrotic core

Coronary plaques frequently contain tissue components with different acoustical characteristics. The IVUS image of mixed plaques can vary between echolucent and echodense, with and without shadowing.

The finding of a hypodense area separated from the lumen by a hyperdense 'cap', as shown in this figure, is often assumed to be evidence of a necrotic core with a fibrous cap. However, most fibrous caps are too thin to be resolved by IVUS and a zone of reduced echogenicity may also be attributable to an intramural hemorrhage, or thrombus.

CHAPTER 5.2.4, REFERENCES 22, 76–78

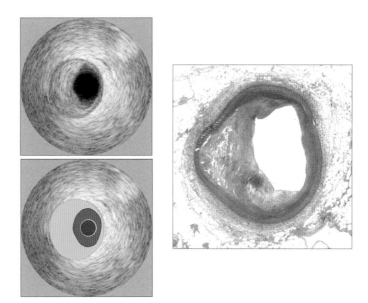

Figure 48   Echogenicity of the necrotic core

The histological correlate of a hypodense region of a plaque, as shown by IVUS (see Figure 47), is often unclear. Similarly, the IVUS appearance of a plaque with a documented necrotic core can also vary.

In this figure, matched histology and IVUS images of a coronary artery examined *ex vivo* are shown. The plaque shows a necrotic core by histology, but appears 'echodense' by IVUS. Histological studies have demonstrated that necrotic lesions often contain microcalcifications mixed with lipid. This may explain the spectrum of echogenicity seen in comparative studies.

CHAPTER 5.2.4, REFERENCES 22, 76–81

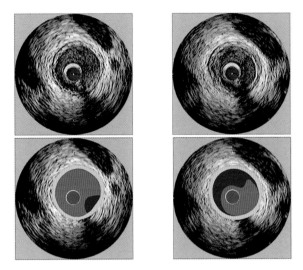

Figure 49   Thrombus

By IVUS, intraluminal thrombus is usually recognized as an intraluminal mass, often with a layered, lobulated, or pedunculated appearance. Thrombi may appear relatively echolucent or have a more variable gray scale. Blood flow in 'microchannels' may also be apparent within some thrombi (Figures 67–70). Stagnant blood flow can simulate a thrombus with a grayish-white accumulation of specular echoes within the vascular lumen. Injection of contrast or saline may disperse stagnant blood and allow differentiation of stasis from thrombosis. However, IVUS is unreliable in differentiating acute thrombi from echolucent plaques.

In this figure, an intraluminal filling defect is shown, which was interpreted as a thrombus.

CHAPTER 5.2.5, REFERENCE 82

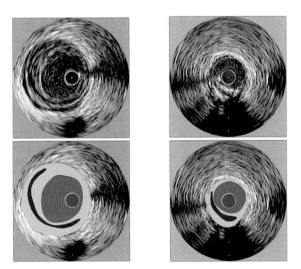

Figure 50   Thrombus/layered plaque

Thrombus often has a layered appearance on IVUS, as shown in this figure. However, the precise pathophysiological correlate of this finding is unclear. It is interesting that recent histological studies describe layered plaques with buried fibrous caps as evidence of previous recurrent events of plaque rupture, thrombosis and healing.

CHAPTER 5.2.5, REFERENCES 82, 179, 180

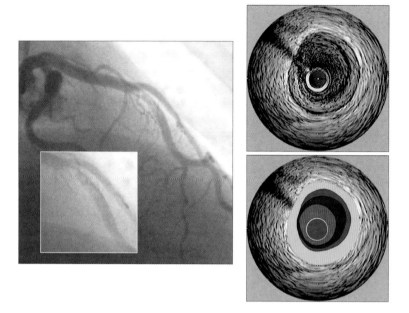

Figure 51   Intracoronary thrombus (1)
A clinical example of angiographically confirmed intracoronary thrombus is shown in this figure. By IVUS, the thrombus has a layered appearance with varying echogenicity, making the assessment of the exact size and the differentiation of the lumen difficult. The angiogram clearly shows the intraluminal filling defect in the mid left anterior descending artery.

CHAPTER 5.2.5, REFERENCES 9, 10, 82

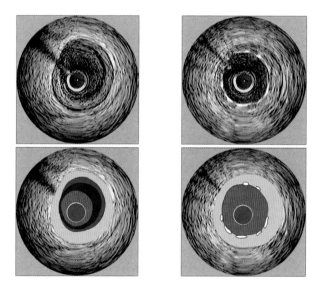

Figure 52   Intracoronary thrombus (2)
The patient was initially treated with an intensive antithrombotic regimen. However, because of repeated ischemic episodes PCI was eventually performed. At the same site as shown in Figure 51, the pre- and post-stenting images are shown.

CHAPTER 5.2.5, REFERENCE 82

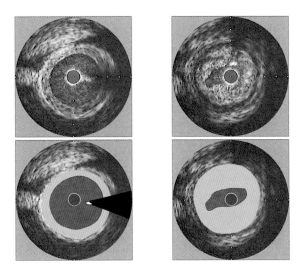

Figure 53   Venous bypass grafts

In vein grafts, wall morphology and plaque characteristics are different from those in native coronary arteries. The wall of the bypass graft is free from the surrounding tissue and has no side-branches. *In situ* vein grafts do not have an EEM. However, vein grafts typically undergo 'arterialization' with morphological changes that include intimal fibrous thickening, medial hypertrophy, and lipid deposition. IVUS measurements, including plaque plus media area and plaque burden, are performed in a similar fashion to those in native coronary disease.

CHAPTER 5.2.7, REFERENCES 9, 10

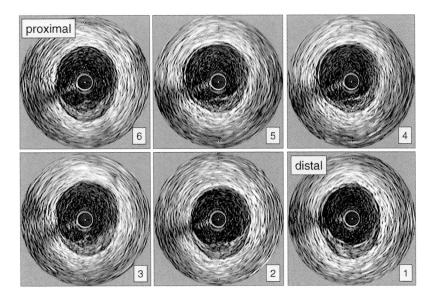

Figure 54   Unstable ('vulnerable') lesions (1)

Most acute coronary syndromes (ACS) are caused by the rupture or erosion of vulnerable plaques. Plaque vulnerability is defined as the tendency of a lesion to rupture or erode, causing subsequent thrombosis, and is therefore a *prospective* definition. The identification of vulnerable lesions *before* rupture is complex and the current role of *in vivo* imaging modalities is still limited.

This figure shows adjacent images from a mildly stenotic lesion with evidence of rupture (panels 3 and 4). This lesion did not cause clinical symptoms. Current prospective IVUS studies describing morphological characteristics of such mildly stenotic lesion may provide insights into the development of unstable (vulnerable) lesions.

CHAPTER 5.2.8, REFERENCES 9, 10, 84–87

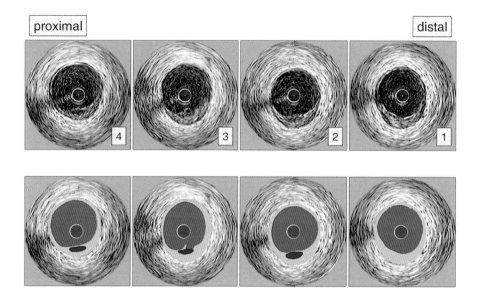

Figure 55   Unstable ('vulnerable') lesions (2)

IVUS cannot *prospectively* identify a plaque as vulnerable. However, there is consistent evidence that echolucent, presumably lipid-laden, and expansive (positive) remodeled plaques more frequently lead to acute coronary syndromes. For these lesions, the terms 'high-risk plaque' and 'thin-cap-necrotic-core atheroma' have been suggested.

This figure illustrates the findings from Figure 54. In the image slices adjacent to the ruptured site (panel 3), the plaque demonstrates echolucency and expansive remodeling.

CHAPTER 5.2.8, REFERENCES 85–96

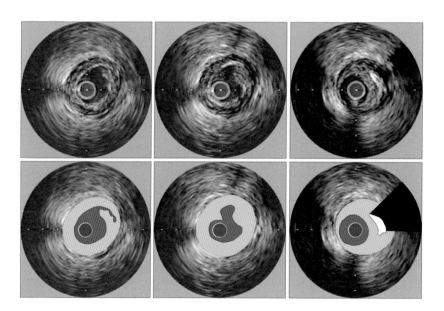

Figure 56   Unstable ('vulnerable') lesions, plaque ulceration and plaque rupture

IVUS criteria for the identification of plaque rupture at culprit lesions have been described. An example of plaque rupture is shown in this figure. Adjacent images demonstrate a plaque cavity in the middle panel and a tissue flap in the left panel.

CHAPTER 5.2.8, REFERENCES 9, 10, 85–87, 184–188

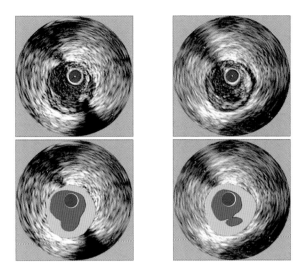

Figure 57   Plaque rupture

Plaque rupture or ulceration is defined by IVUS as a recess in the plaque beginning at the luminal–intimal border. Features supporting intimal disruption are irregular intimal surfaces of ulcerated plaques and visible torn edges in video sequences. Blood flow in the vessel wall cavity is an important criterion and contrast injections may be used to prove and define the communication point. However, ruptured plaques may have a highly variable appearance by IVUS, in particular in the presence of a superimposed thrombus, which is a hallmark of ruptured lesions in histological studies.

This figure shows a ruptured plaque with a remaining cavity at the 6 o'clock position.

CHAPTER 5.2.8, REFERENCES 9, 10, 85–87, 184, 185

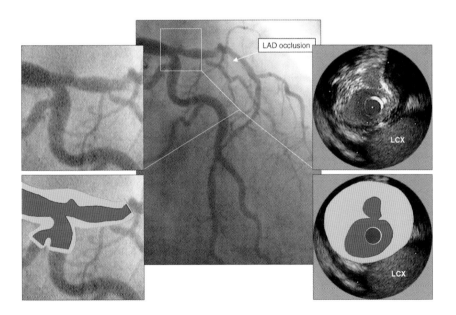

Figure 58   Plaque rupture: comparison IVUS and angiography

This illustration demonstrates a cavity in the vessel wall of the ostial left anterior descending artery identified with IVUS and angiography. The angiographic appearance of these cavities is a focal area of bulging of the lumen. The size of the plaque is not directly seen with angiography. The patient presented with an acute myocardial infarction secondary to the occlusive lesion of the mid left anterior descending artery.

CHAPTER 5.2.8, REFERENCES 9, 10, 85–87, 184, 185

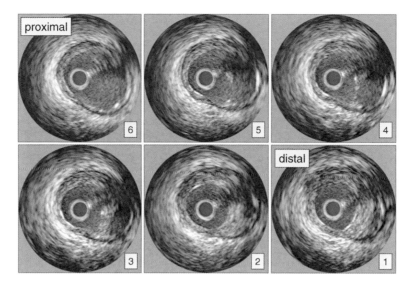

Figure 59   Plaque rupture with large cavity (1)

An example of plaque rupture with large cavity is shown in this figure. Sequential images from a pullback demonstrate an eccentric plaque with a large cavity. In the video sequences, blood flow could clearly be seen in the cavity, confirming the communication between lumen and cavity. An echodense narrow structure separates the cavity from the lumen in panel 4 and could represent remnants of the fibrous cap.

CHAPTER 5.2.8, REFERENCES 9, 10, 86, 87

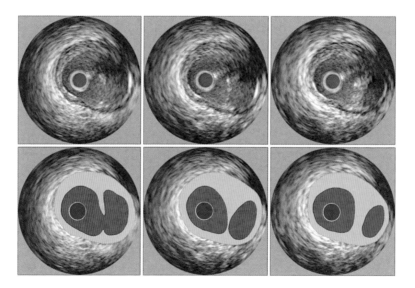

Figure 60   Plaque rupture with large cavity (2)

The illustration of Figure 59 demonstrates the large cavity in the vessel wall. It is unclear why the cavity is not filled by thrombus, which is one of the characteristics of ruptured plaques in histological studies. It is also not known if such a lesion represents an active lesion with high risk of subsequent thrombosis or if such lesions could be stable remnants of past rupture.

CHAPTER 5.2.8, REFERENCES 85, 86, 179–181, 186

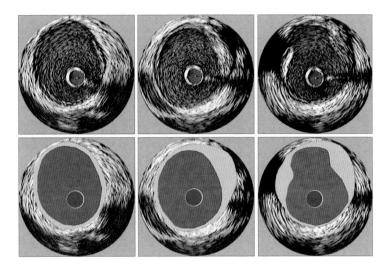

Figure 61   Healed plaque rupture? (1)
Recent histological studies demonstrate that plaque rupture is a frequent event and often clinically asymptomatic. The IVUS examination of vessel segments not related to acute coronary events occasionally shows cavities in the vessel wall, as shown in this figure.

It is an attractive hypothesis that they could be remnants of healed plaque rupture, but this is not proven by histological studies or serial *in vivo* imaging.

CHAPTER 5.2.8, REFERENCES 9, 10, 86, 87, 179–181, 184–188

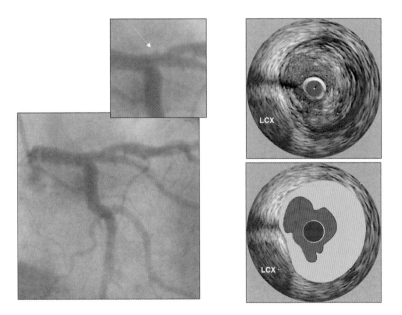

Figure 62   Healed plaque rupture? (2)
The figure demonstrates angiographic and IVUS images of an asymptomatic patient with a cavity in the vessel wall at the proximal left anterior descending artery. The cavities seen on the IVUS image at the 11 o'clock position correspond to the focal bulge at the proximal left anterior descending artery (arrow) (compare with Figure 58).

CHAPTER 5.2.8, REFERENCES 9, 10, 85–87, 179–181, 184, 185

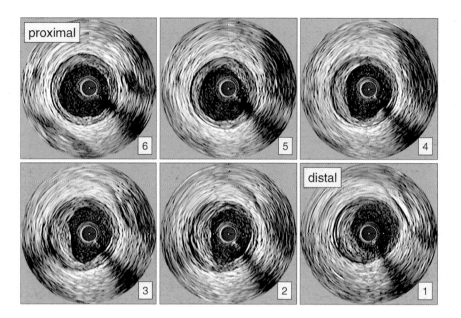

Figure 63   Healed plaque rupture? (3)
A more subtle example of such a cavity is shown in this figure. Sequential images from a pullback show evidence of a cavity at the 7 o'clock position.

CHAPTER 5.2.8, REFERENCES 9, 10, 86, 87, 179–181, 184–188

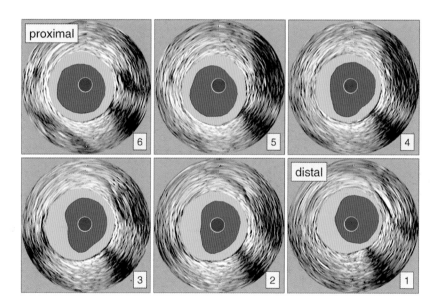

Figure 64   Healed plaque rupture? (4)
The color illustration of the previous figure demonstrates the asymmetric shape of the lumen with the cavity at the 7 o'clock position.

CHAPTER 5.2.8, REFERENCES 9, 10, 86, 87, 179–181, 184–188

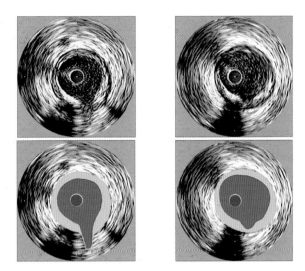

Figure 65   Differential diagnosis of plaque rupture: vessel branch
Importantly, a side-branch entering the main vessel can appear as a plaque cavity on individual still images. The evaluation of adjacent images can differentiate these findings and should always be performed carefully.

CHAPTER 5.2.8, REFERENCES 9, 10, 86, 87

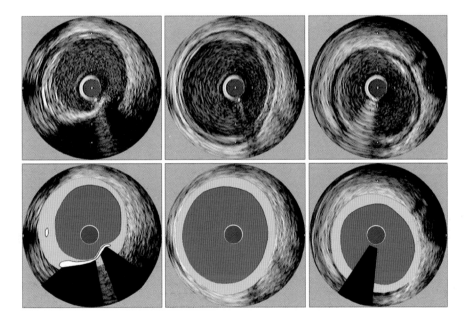

Figure 66   Coronary aneurysm
A true coronary aneurysm describes a vessel expansion involving all layers of the vessel wall. A frequently used definition requires that the EEM and lumen are > 50% larger than those of the proximal reference segment. Of note, expansive (positive) arterial remodeling and focal aneurysms may be related processes on a spectrum of disease manifestations.
A pseudoaneurysm is defined as a disruption of the EEM, usually observed after intervention (see Figures 99 and 100).

CHAPTER 5.2.9, REFERENCES 9, 10, 97

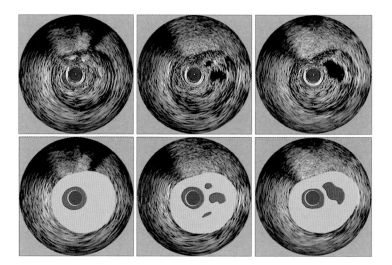

Figure 67   True versus false lumen? (1)

It is sometimes difficult to differentiate true versus false vessel lumen. Possible hints are that a true lumen is surrounded by the vessel intima, media, and adventitia.

This figure shows images from a patient who presented with stable angina. In the left panel, a severe stenosis is demonstrated. It is unclear if the hypodense areas in the plaque (middle and right images) represent a false lumen secondary to recanalization of a thrombosed true lumen.

CHAPTERS 5.2.5 AND 5.2.9, REFERENCES 9, 10

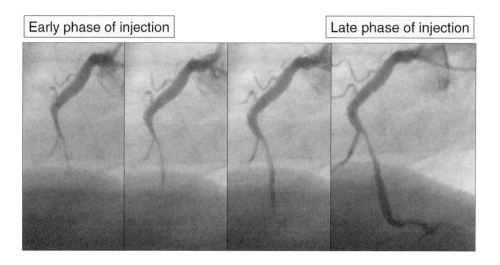

Figure 68   True versus false lumen? (2)

In this figure, several images of the corresponding angiogram, obtained during several phases of contrast injection, are shown. The severe lesion of the right coronary artery is obvious, confirming the IVUS findings. An explanation of the additional IVUS findings was not found.

CHAPTERS 5.2.5 AND 5.2.9, REFERENCES 9, 10

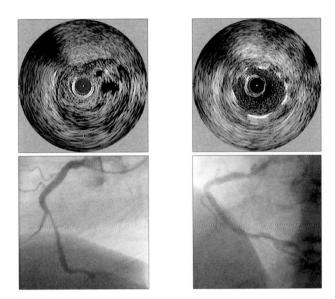

Figure 69: True versus false lumen? (3)

PCI of the right coronary artery lesion was performed. In this figure, the pre- and post-interventional angiogram and IVUS are shown together.

CHAPTERS 5.2.5 AND 5.2.9, REFERENCES 9, 10

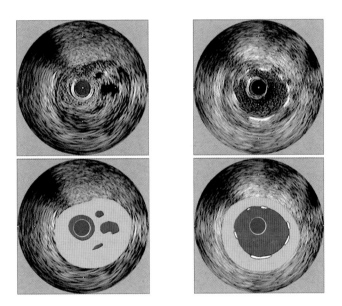

Figure 70   True versus false lumen? (4)

The color-illustrated pre- and post-interventional IVUS images are shown here. Despite careful analysis, the pre-interventional anatomy remained unclear but was thought to represent false channels in a thrombosed true lumen.

CHAPTERS 5.2.5 AND 5.2.9, REFERENCES 9, 10

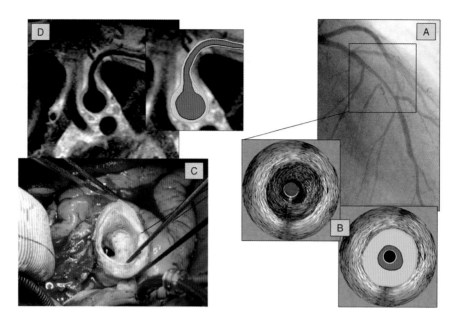

Figure 71   Coronary arteritis

This figure shows the post-procedural angiogram and IVUS (panels A and B) from a young patient, who presented with an acute myocardial infarction in 2001. A stent was placed in the left anterior descending artery. The smooth narrowing on the angiogram proximal to a stent corresponds to a large concentric plaque burden, as demonstrated by IVUS.

Two years later, the patient underwent coronary artery bypass graft for progression of coronary disease. The ascending aorta showed signs of significant thickening and inflammation and was replaced during the surgery (panel C). The pathology was consistent with Takayasu arteritis.

The postoperative magnetic resonance imaging scan shows evidence of mild wall thickening in the aortic arch distal to the grafted ascending aorta (panel D).

It remained unclear if the IVUS finding in 2001 represented inflammatory wall thickening of the coronary arteries.

CHAPTER 5.2.9, REFERENCES 9, 10, 98

Established clinical applications

Established clinical indications to perform IVUS are the evaluation of unclear angiographic finding, the guidance of percutaneous coronary intervention (PCI), and the assessment of transplant vasculopathy. More recently, IVUS is performed in serial studies examining the progression/regression of coronary arterial disease (Chapter 7).

CHAPTER 6

ASSESSMENT OF ANGIOGRAPHICALLY INDETERMINATE LESIONS

Angiographically normal coronary arteries are encountered in 10–15% of patients undergoing catheterization for suspected coronary disease. IVUS commonly detects occult disease in these patients.

Certain lesion subsets elude accurate angiographic characterization, despite thorough examination using multiple radiographic projections. These angiographically ambiguous lesions include lesions with intermediate stenotic severity, ostial stenosis, left main stem lesions, and dissections after coronary angioplasty.

IVUS is frequently employed to examine lesions with the above characteristics, in some cases providing additional evidence useful in determining whether the stenosis is clinically significant. In other clinical situations, it may be preferable to obtain hemodynamic information.

CHAPTER 6.1, REFERENCES 99–103

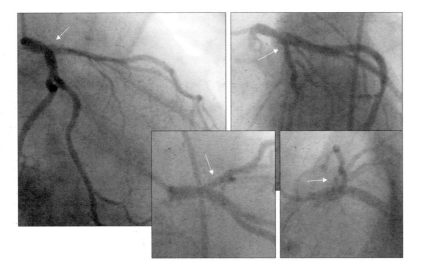

Figure 72   Angiographically indeterminate lesion (1.1)
Figures 72–76 show angiographic and IVUS images of a hazy proximal left anterior descending artery (LAD) lesion. The patient had classic exertional angina and a stress test was consistent with anterior wall ischemia. Despite evaluation in several angiographic planes, the angiographic assessment was incomplete and the stenosis severity of the proximal LAD lesion remained unclear. A physiological assessment (fractional-flow reserve (FFR) = 0.85) was not consistent with a hemodynamically significant lesion. The operator decided to perform IVUS.

CHAPTER 6.1, REFERENCES 99–103

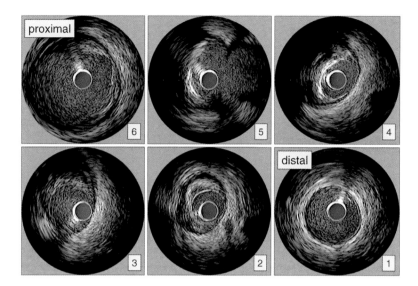

Figure 73   Angiographically indeterminate lesion (1.2)

Intravascular ultrasound of the proximal LAD demonstrated a relatively tight stenosis (panels 2 and 4). The minimal luminal area at site 2 was less than 4 mm², which is a frequently used IVUS criteria of significant stenosis. The proximal LAD demonstrates heavy calcification (panels 4 and 5).

CHAPTER 6.1, REFERENCES 99–103

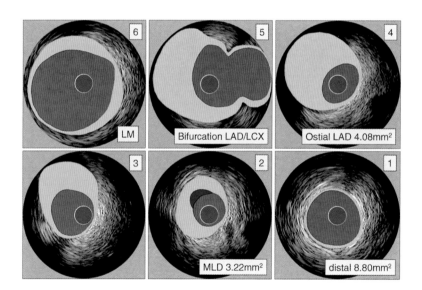

Figure 74   Angiographically indeterminate lesion (1.3)

The intravascular ultrasound findings are illustrated in this figure. The tight stenosis at sites 2 and 4 is obvious. The large plaque burden at site 4 is also noteworthy.

CHAPTER 6.1, REFERENCES 99–103

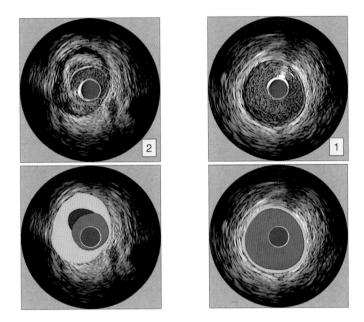

Figure 75   Angiographically indeterminate lesion (1.4)
The findings at the worst lesion site and the distal reference site are compared in this figure. Based on this IVUS information, PCI was performed.

CHAPTER 6.1, REFERENCES: 99–103

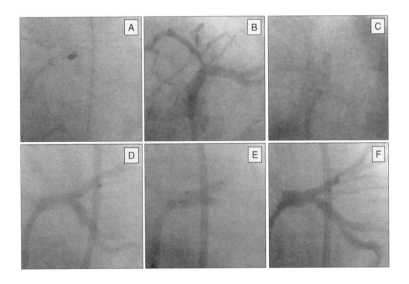

Figure 76   Angiographically indeterminate lesion (1.5)
The PCI included initial rotablation (panels A and B) and subsequent stenting (panel C) of the proximal LAD. Plaque shift at the LAD/LCX bifurcation during the inflation of the LAD stent caused a new obstruction of the LCX ostium (panel D). Therefore, a simultaneous balloon inflation in the LAD and LCX (kissing balloon technique)(panel E) was performed. It is remarkable but not surprising that the plaque shift occurred at a site with large plaque burden (Figures 73 and 74, panel 4).

CHAPTER 6.1, REFERENCES 99–103

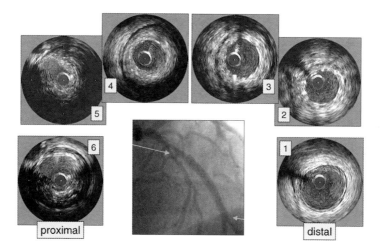

Figure 77 Angiographically indeterminate lesion (2.1)

Figures 77–79 are an example of the disparities that exist between angiography and ultrasound after percutaneous coronary interventions. The post-interventional shape of the lumen may be extremely complex, with plaque fissures or deep wall dissections.

The figure shows the angiogram and IVUS images after PTCA and stenting of a mid LAD lesion in the setting of an acute myocardial infarction. The coronary segment proximal to the stent, where balloon inflations have been performed, is angiographically not clearly defined and appears 'hazy'. IVUS was performed to further evaluate the anatomy (panels 5 and 6).

CHAPTER 6.1, REFERENCES 99–103

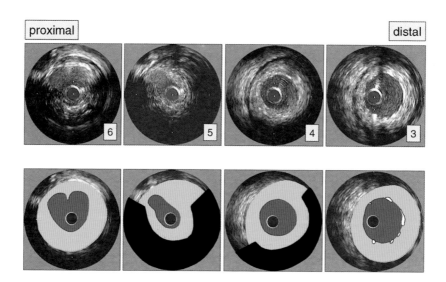

Figure 78 Angiographically indeterminate lesion (2.2)

The illustrations of the IVUS images (panels 3–6 from Figure 77) demonstrate the expanded and well-opposed stent struts in panel 3. However, a tight, complex stenosis is documented proximal to the stent in panel 5.

The luminal area at site 5 was less than 4 mm², which is a frequently used IVUS criterion of significant stenosis.

CHAPTER 6.1, REFERENCES 99–103

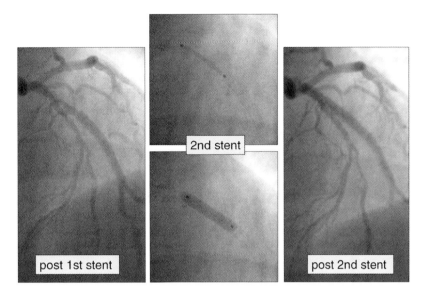

Figure 79   Angiographically indeterminate lesion (2.3)
Based on these findings, an additional stent was deployed proximal to the first stent with minimal overlap. The excellent angiographic results are shown in this figure.

CHAPTER 6.1, REFERENCES 99–103

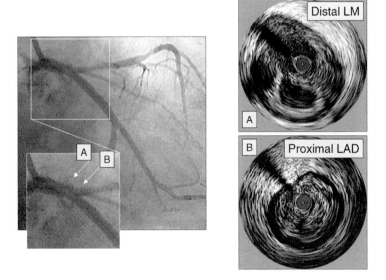

Figure 80   Angiographically indeterminate lesion: left main disease (1)
Assessment of left main (LM) disease by angiography represents a particularly difficult clinical problem. Aortic cusp opacification or 'streaming' of contrast may obscure the ostium, the short length of the vessel may leave no normal segment for comparison, and the distal left main artery may be concealed by the LAD/LCX bifurcation. In most cases, careful angiographic assessment can establish the diagnosis.

In selected cases, IVUS can provide additional information. For a complete interrogation of the LM it is important that a slow pullback of the ultrasound transducer is performed with the guiding catheter disengaged from the LM ostium.

In this figure, the angiogram shows a contrast-filled structure in the distal LM (site A), with an additional hazy lesion in the ostium of the LAD (site B).

IVUS demonstrates a severe ostial lesion of the LAD (panel B). In the distal LM, an eccentric plaque with a large cavity, which is connected to the lumen, is demonstrated (panel A).

CHAPTER 6.1.1, REFERENCES 104–106

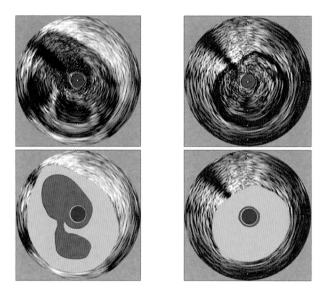

Figure 81   Angiographically indeterminate lesion: left main disease (2)
This illustration of the findings in Figure 80 demonstrates the severe ostial lesion of the LAD (right panels) and the cavity in the distal LM (left panels). This plaque cavity has probably developed after lesion rupture.

CHAPTER 6.1.1, REFERENCES 104–106

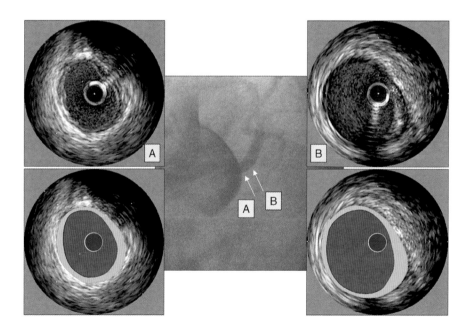

Figure 82   Left main coronary artery: ostial narrowing
The assessment of the LM ostium is often particularly challenging. Importantly, recent IVUS studies have demonstrated physiological, non-atherosclerotic ostial LM narrowing. This phenomenon has also been called 'reverse tapering' and cannot be differentiated from an ostial atherosclerotic stenosis by angiography alone.

CHAPTER 6.1.1, REFERENCE 106

Assessment of transplant vasculopathy

An important application of IVUS is the diagnosis and serial observation of transplant vasculopathy. Coronary transplant vasculopathy represents the major cause of death after the first year following transplantation. Its development is often clinically silent because the transplanted heart is denervated. Ischemia by functional testing does not usually occur until the disease is advanced.

Surveillance angiography identifies focal stenotic disease in 10–20% of patients at 1 year and 50% by 5 years after transplantation. However, it underestimates the diffuse nature of transplant vasculopathy.

IVUS allows the assessment of early plaque accumulation before luminal stenosis develops and has emerged as the optimal method for early detection.

CHAPTER 6.2, REFERENCES 107–126

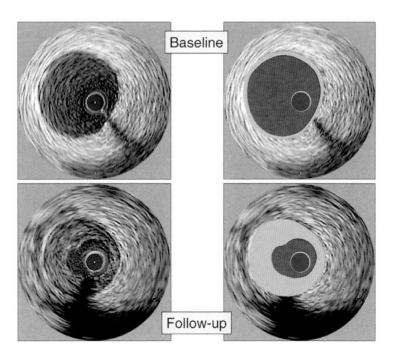

Figure 83 Transplant vasculopathy
Using IVUS, evidence of vasculopathy (defined as abnormal intimal thickening > 0.5 mm) is detected in 50% of patients by 1 year. Transplant vasculopathy, which develops after transplantation, must be differentiated from donor disease that is transplanted into the recipient.

Despite the young donor age, conventional atherosclerosis is frequently present in donor hearts. In a study from our group, atherosclerotic lesions were detected in 56% of patients at a mean donor age of 32 years[112].

In this figure, serial images at the same site in a vessel segment are shown at baseline (upper panels) and at 1-year follow-up (lower panels). The interval development of significant intimal thickening is clearly shown. More recent IVUS studies of transplant vasculopathy utilize a volumetric analysis of intimal changes (see Chapter 7.2).

CHAPTER 6.2, REFERENCES 118–124

Interventional applications

Although IVUS has played a pivotal role in understanding the effects of interventional devices, the precise clinical role for ultrasound during intervention has, for the most part, not been well defined in large-scale clinical trials. It would be beyond the scope of this Atlas to discuss specific details of interventional indications. However, the pertinent literature is summarized in the Manual. The following slides demonstrate the interaction between percutaneous coronary intervention and plaque characteristics.

CHAPTER 6.3, REFERENCES 88, 90–93, 102, 103, 127–129

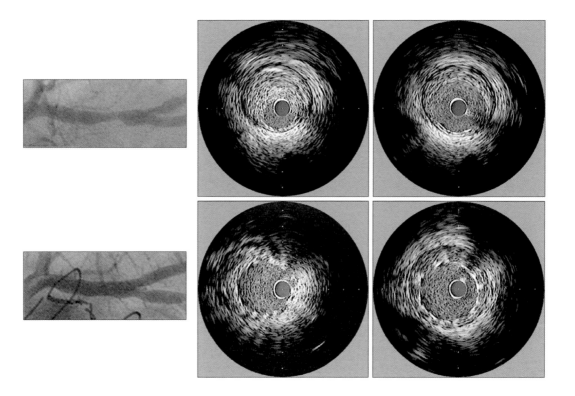

Figure 84　Vessel wall characteristics and coronary stent expansion (1)
Recent clinical IVUS studies describe how pre-interventional plaque characteristics, including plaque echogenicity and remodeling, determine the revascularization rate of the target lesion.

　　This and the next figure show the stent expansion at the site of a tight lesion and the mildly diseased reference site. The images demonstrate how plaque size, composition, and eccentricity influence the extent of stent expansion.

CHAPTER 6.3, REFERENCES 88, 90–93, 127–129

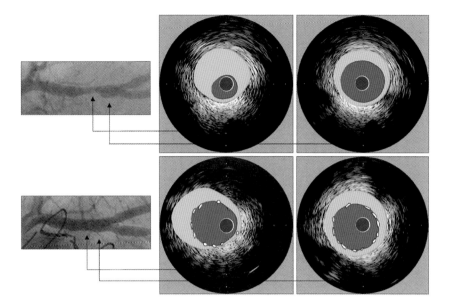

Figure 85   Vessel wall characteristics and coronary stent expansion (2)
The illustration of the previous figure shows the more eccentric residual plaque distribution at the lesion site (left panels). In contrast, the stented reference lumen is more circular and symmetric (right panels).

CHAPTER 6.3, REFERENCES 88, 90–93, 127–129

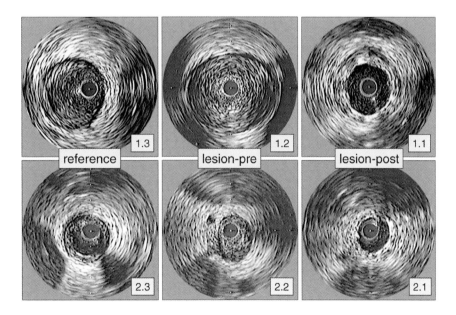

Figure 86   Plaque burden and coronary stenting (1)
This and the next figure illustrate the complex interaction of plaque burden, remodeling and lumen size during intervention.

In the upper row, the reference site (panel 1.3), pre-interventional lesion site (panel 1.2), and post-interventional lesion site (panel 1.1) of a lesion with a large plaque burden and expansive remodeling are shown.

In the lower row, the reference site (panel 2.3), pre-interventional lesion site (panel 2.2), and post-interventional lesion site (panel 2.1) of a lesion with a small plaque burden and constrictive remodeling are shown.

CHAPTER 6.3.1, REFERENCES 90–93, 127–129

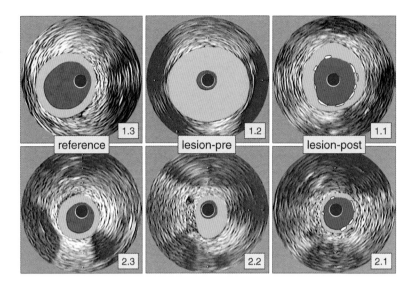

Figure 87 Plaque burden and coronary stenting (2)
The illustrated images demonstrate the large plaque burden with expansive remodeling at the lesion site in the upper row (panel 1.2), and a smaller plaque burden with constrictive remodeling at the lesion site in the lower row (panel 2.2). Despite the large differences in plaque size at the lesion site, the luminal dimensions (and hence the angiographic appearance) of these lesions are similar. However, it is conceivable that the responses to PCI are different.

CHAPTER 6.3.1, REFERENCES 90–93, 127–129

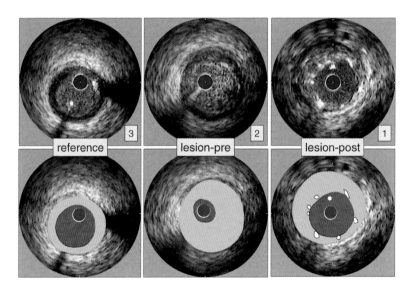

Figure 88 Expansive remodeling and coronary stenting
This figure shows a lesion with expansive (positive) remodeling at the lesion site before and after stenting.

Recent studies describe that PTCA is associated with a higher target lesion revascularization rate in expansive (positive) remodeled lesions. However, in other studies, this relationship was not found after stenting.

CHAPTER 6.3.1, REFERENCES 127–129

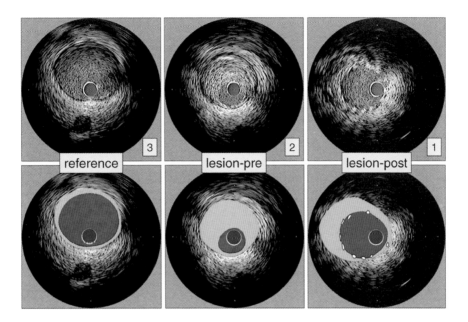

Figure 89   Constrictive remodeling and coronary stenting
In contrast to Figure 88, this figure shows a lesion with constrictive (negative) remodeling at the lesion site before and after stenting. According to the afore-mentioned studies, constrictive (negative) remodeling is associated with decrease target lesion revascularization rate after PTCA.

CHAPTER 6.3.1, REFERENCES 127–129

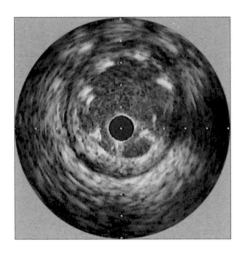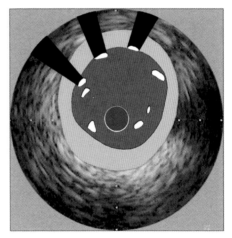

Figure 90   Coronary stenting: unopposed stent struts
IVUS imaging has played an important role in understanding the benefits of stent therapy.

Columbo and colleagues demonstrated that stent deployment with conventional balloon pressures resulted in a high incidence of incomplete stent expansion. Subsequent studies demonstrated that intravascular ultrasound-guided high-pressure dilatation achieved full expansion and complete stent apposition in a large percentage of patients, using only aspirin and ticlopidine after the procedure.

Larger trials demonstrated the safety of stent implantation using high pressures and antiplatelet therapy alone (without IVUS guidance). Consistent with these later trials, IVUS is not routinely used for stent optimization today, although there is great variability in its application from center to center.

CHAPTER 6.3.3, REFERENCES 148–154

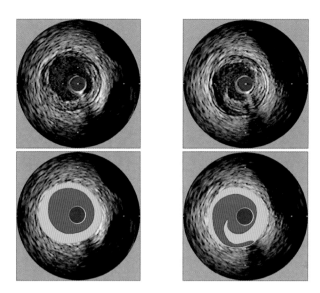

Figure 91   Complications of PCI: dissection
IVUS is commonly employed to identify dissections and other complications after intervention.

In this figure, a relatively large dissection flap is seen after PCI at the site of balloon inflation (6 o'clock position in the right panel).

CHAPTER 6.3.4, REFERENCES 51–53, 134, 155

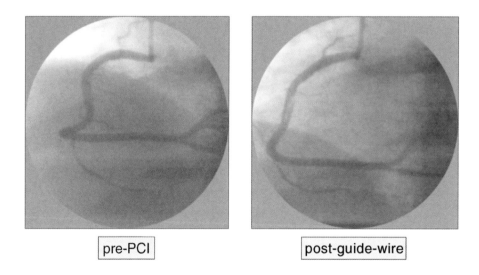

Figure 92   Complications of IVUS/PCI: dissection (1)
The safety of intracoronary ultrasound is well documented. Major complications, including dissection or vessel closure, are uncommon (less than < 0.5%) and typically occur in patients undergoing intervention rather than diagnostic imaging.

Despite this favorable safety profile, subselective coronary instrumentation always carries a potential risk of significant vessel injury and should only be performed by operators experienced in diagnostic and interventional therapeutic intracoronary catheter manipulation.

In the following figures (Figures 92–95) a case of dissection after diagnostic IVUS is demonstrated. The angiogram after insertion of the guide-wire shows an intravascular filling defect in the mid-RCA.

CHAPTERS 1.3.1 AND 6.3.4, REFERENCES 11, 12

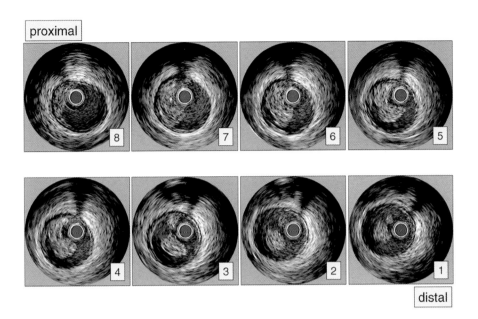

Figure 93   Complications of IVUS/PCI: dissection (2)
Adjacent IVUS images at the lesion site are shown. The images confirm a intraluminal filling defect consistent with a dissection and superimposed thrombus. The flap/ thrombus appears as a free-floating structure in panels 1–3 and opposed to the wall in panels 4–7.

CHAPTERS 1.3.1 AND 6.3.4, REFERENCES 9–12

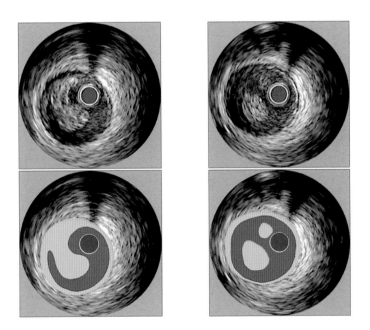

Figure 94   Complications of IVUS/PCI: dissection (3)
The IVUS findings are illustrated in this figure. The distal end of the dissection flap/thrombus is surrounded by blood flow, giving the appearance of a free-floating structure.

CHAPTERS 1.3.1 AND 6.3.4, REFERENCES 9–12

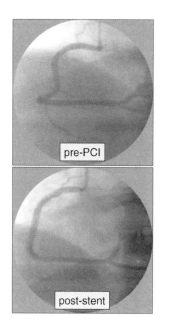
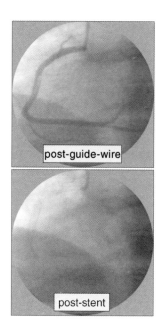

Figure 95   Complications of IVUS/PCI: dissection (4)

Percutaneous coronary intervention was performed. The pre- and post-interventional angiograms are shown. The dissection flap was opposed to the wall by a coronary stent.

CHAPTERS 1.3.1 AND 6.3.4, REFERENCES 11, 12

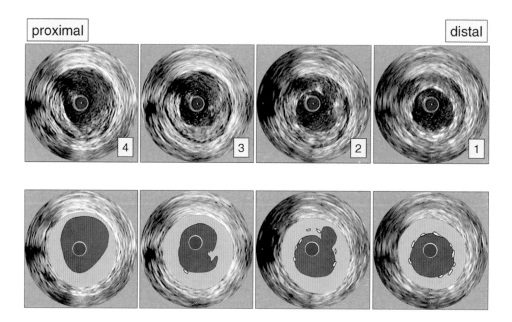

Figure 96   Dissection after stenting (1)

In this figure, post-interventional IVUS images of a small dissection at the proximal edge of a stent are seen immediately after stent deployment.

CHAPTER 6.3.4, REFERENCES 51–53, 134, 155

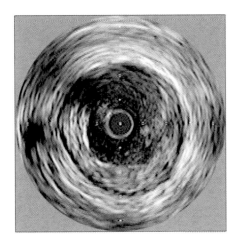
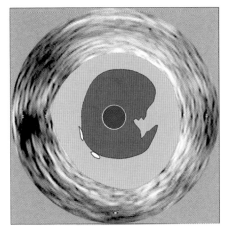

Figure 97   Dissection after stenting (2)
The enlarged illustration of panel 3 from the previous figure clearly shows a small dissection flap at the 3 o'clock position. The struts at 7 o'clock are the proximal end of the deployed stent.

CHAPTER 6.3.4, REFERENCES 51–53, 134, 155

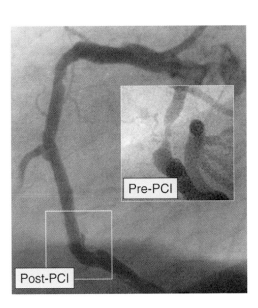
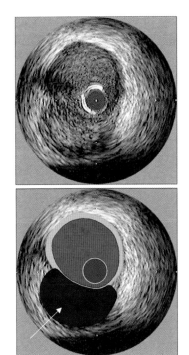

Figure 98   Intramural hematoma post-PCI
An intramural hematoma is defined as an accumulation of blood within the medial space, displacing the internal elastic membrane inward and EEM outward. The entry and/or exit points may be observed.

In this example, an intramural hematoma (arrow) has developed after PTCA of a tight RCA lesion.

CHAPTER 6.3.4, REFERENCES 9, 10, 51–53, 134, 155

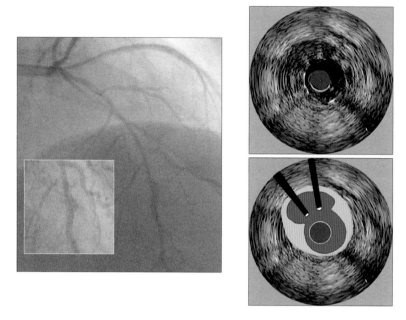

Figure 99   Chronic coronary arterial wall dissection behind stent (1)

These images were obtained during repeat angiography several weeks after stent placement in the mid LAD. The angiography is consistent with a spiral dissection, which is confirmed by IVUS. The subacute dissection is located behind the stent struts.

CHAPTER 6.3.4, REFERENCES 51–53, 134, 155

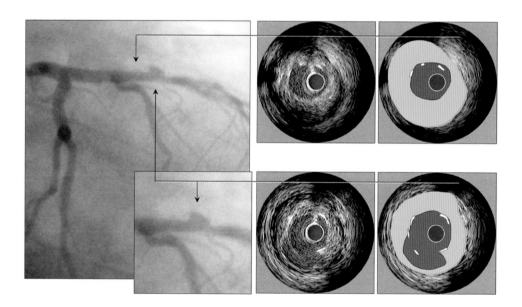

Figure 100 Chronic coronary arterial wall dissection behind stent (2)

These images show the angiogram and the IVUS images of another patient, who developed a chronic dissection at the proximal edge of a previously placed stent.

The angiography shows a contrast pool outside the lumen, consistent with a dissection. The IVUS images demonstrate that the dissection is located behind the stent struts.

CHAPTER 6.3.4, REFERENCES 51–53, 134, 155

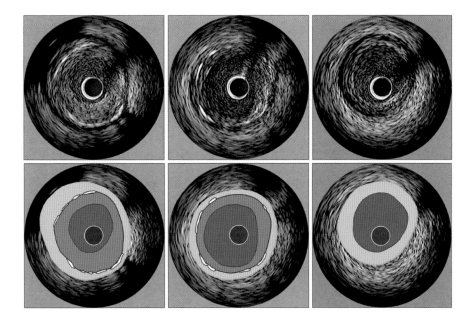

Figure 101 Complications of PCI: in-stent restenosis (ISR)

Unlike the restenotic response after angioplasty or atherectomy, which is a mixture of constrictive (negative) arterial remodeling and neointimal growth, in-stent restenosis is primarily due to neointimal proliferation.

The intimal hyperplasia characteristic of early in-stent restenosis often exhibits very low echogenicity. Appropriate system settings are critical to avoid suppressing this relative non-echogenic material. The intimal hyperplasia of late in-stent restenosis often appears more echogenic.

CHAPTER 6.3.5, REFERENCES 73, 83, 156–161

Evolving clinical and research applications

Exciting new applications for IVUS are the assessment and serial observation of plaque burden and mechanisms of atherosclerosis development, including plaque stability/vulnerability.

These evolving clinical and research applications, summarized as 'atherosclerosis imaging', have already enhanced our understanding of atherosclerotic plaque development and will likely have an important impact on coronary artery disease prevention.

CHAPTER 7 REFERENCES 29–31, 68, 69, 186, 189

ASSESSMENT OF PLAQUE VULNERABILITY

Rupture or superficial erosion of vulnerable coronary plaques with subsequent thrombosis represents the principal pathophysiology underlying most acute coronary syndromes. Plaque vulnerability describes a temporary activated state of atherosclerotic plaques, leading to a higher risk of plaque rupture and thrombosis. Most vulnerable plaques stabilize either without rupture or after episodes of rupture and fibrosis, and only in a few cases do rupture and thrombosis lead to vessel occlusion and acute coronary syndromes.

The *in vivo* identification of vulnerable plaques before rupture would allow the development of interventions directed at plaque stabilization. However, because vulnerable lesions are a temporary stage in plaque development, their temporal and spatial distribution in the entire coronary tree is highly dynamic and dependent on the clinical situation.

The assessment of plaque vulnerability using IVUS therefore faces two challenges: the morphologic characterization of *focal* lesions but also the assessment of the *systemic* disease process.

Currently, a reliable identification of vulnerable plaque before rupture is not possible with IVUS.

CHAPTER 7.1, REFERENCES 29, 170–189

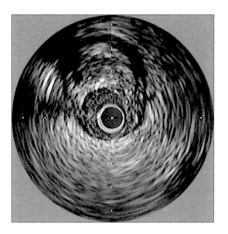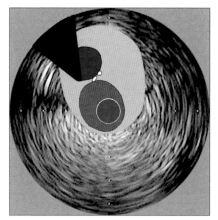

Figure 102 Plaque vulnerability: necrotic core

IVUS studies have compared plaque characteristics in severely stenotic culprit lesions of patients with stable and unstable coronary syndromes. Plaque echolucency, which correlates with the lipid content of plaques, has been associated with the clinical presentation of unstable angina.

This figure illustrates a plaque with heterogeneous composition showing a prominent echolucent core and an echogenic border structure at the lumen– intima interface. It is not completely clear if this morphology reflects a necrotic core and fibrous cap, which are the histological characteristic of vulnerable lesions. It is important to consider that most fibrous caps are too thin to be resolved by IVUS and a zone of reduced echogenicity may also be attributable to an intramural hemorrhage, or thrombus. Therefore reliable identification of 'vulnerable' lesions is currently not possible.

CHAPTER 7.1, REFERENCES 76–78, 85, 88–92, 186

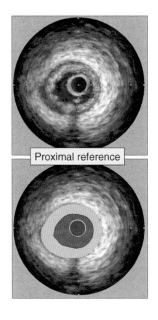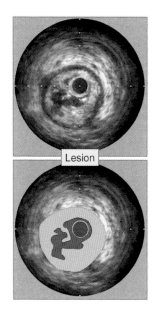

Proximal reference

Lesion

Figure 103 Plaque vulnerability and expansive remodeling

Recent histological and IVUS studies describe an association between clinical presentation and remodeling of the culprit lesion. In patients presenting with unstable angina or acute myocardial infarction, expansive (positive) remodeling is significantly more prevalent than in patients presenting with stable angina. The outward remodeled lesion sites typically harbor significantly larger plaques and are characterized by an intense inflammatory response.

In these images from a patient presenting with an acute myocardial infarction, the lesion site demonstrates expansive (positive) remodeling and a ruptured plaque.

CHAPTER 7.1, REFERENCES 64, 65, 91–95, 190, 191

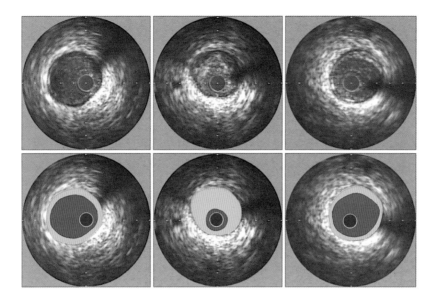

Figure 104 Constrictive remodeling and stable clinical presentation

Conversely, lesions causing stable angina are frequently characterized by constrictive (negative) remodeling. It has been proposed that the fibrotic changes associated with negative remodeling may increase internal plaque resistance to rupture.

CHAPTER 7.1, REFERENCES 64, 65, 203, 204

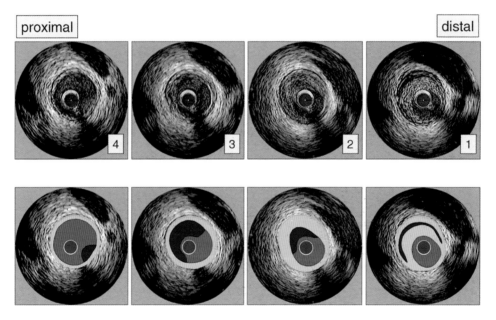

Figure 105 Plaque vulnerability: rupture and thrombosis

Most acute coronary syndromes are initiated by plaque rupture or erosion of mildly stenotic lesions. The size and stability of the developing superimposed thrombus determine the clinical fate of the patient. A large occlusive thrombus causes acute myocardial infarction or sudden cardiac death (SCD). A small thrombus may initiate a form of plaque healing and may frequently be asymptomatic.

The identification of thrombus with IVUS is unreliable, because of varying echogenicity. It is therefore likely that the identification of plaque rupture with IVUS is limited in the presence of a superimposed thrombus.

In these images of a patient presenting with an acute coronary syndrome, a plaque with areas of low echogenicity is shown. The layered appearance evident in panel 1 is further evidence for thrombus.

CHAPTER 7.1, REFERENCES 82, 179, 180

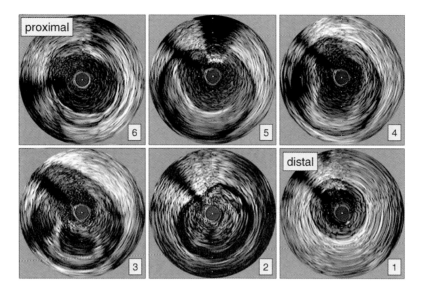

Figure 106 Plaque vulnerability: rupture of culprit lesion (1)
Plaque rupture at culprit lesion sites causing acute coronary syndromes has been well described in histological studies. However, the temporal relationship between acute event and morphological findings with imaging modalities is not well understood.

IVUS pullback through diseased segments often reveals plaque cavities. Although it is generally accepted that these cavities reflect the remnants of ruptured plaques, the absence of thrombus is remarkable. However, histological studies have described that finding previously.

In this and the following figure, a plaque cavity in the distal left main artery in conjunction with a severely stenotic lesion in the proximal left anterior descending artery is shown.

CHAPTER 7.1, REFERENCES 85–87, 179, 180, 181, 186

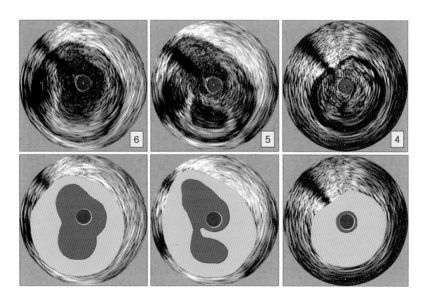

Figure 107 Plaque vulnerability: rupture of culprit lesion (2)
The illustration of the previous figure clearly shows the large plaque burden of the highly stenotic lesion in the proximal left anterior descending artery (panel 4) and the plaque cavity in the distal left main artery (panel 5).

CHAPTER 7.1, REFERENCES 9, 10, 85–87, 179, 180, 181, 186

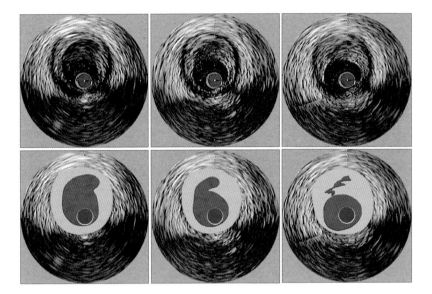

Figure 108 Plaque vulnerability: rupture of mildly stenotic lesions

Most acute coronary syndromes are initiated after sudden changes of mildly stenotic plaques, which did not cause prior symptoms. Therefore prospective examination of mildly stenotic lesions would be the most promising approach in identifying morphological characteristics associated with future plaque rupture and clinical events.

In this figure, a moderate stenotic lesion with plaque rupture is shown. This lesion did not cause clinical symptoms.

CHAPTER 7.1.2, REFERENCES 84, 96, 176, 179, 180, 186

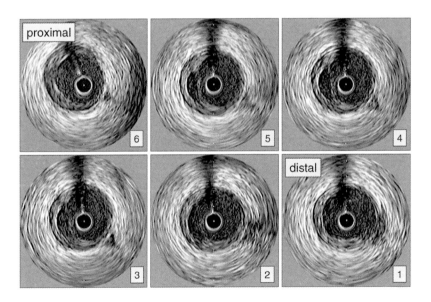

Figure 109 Plaque vulnerability: rupture distant of culprit lesion (1)

Recent studies describe that most episodes of plaque rupture are clinically silent and only occasionally result in an acute coronary syndrome.

In this figure, an example of a mildly stenotic lesion with evidence of plaque rupture is shown. The lesion did not cause clinical symptoms.

CHAPTER 7.1.2, REFERENCES 85, 179–188

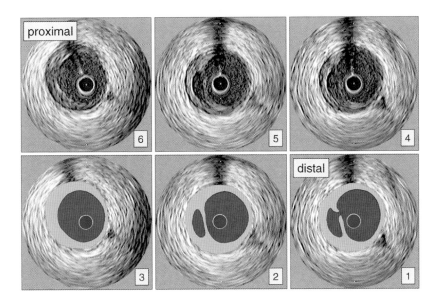

Figure 110 Plaque vulnerability: rupture distant of culprit lesion (2)
Angioscopic, angiographic and IVUS studies have demonstrated lesions with characteristics of plaque vulnerability or rupture at sites other than the culprit lesion in patients presenting with acute coronary syndromes.
The illustration of these images from the previous figure clearly show the site of rupture.

CHAPTER 7.1.2, REFERENCES 85, 179–188

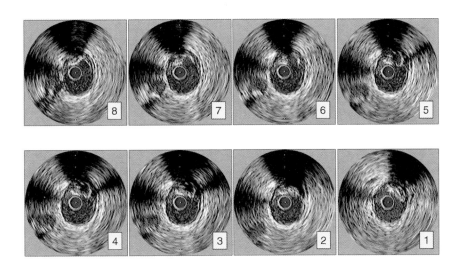

Figure 111 Plaque vulnerability: rupture and calcification (1)
The relation between plaque vulnerability, rupture and calcification is complex and only partially understood. Large calcifications may be associated with stable lesions. In contrast, microcalcifications are frequently found in lipid-rich necrotic core areas of unstable plaques and may not be well reflected in IVUS images.
An example of a calcified lesion with an adjacent prominent plaque cavity is shown in this figure.

CHAPTERS 5.2.3 AND 7.1, REFERENCES 80, 81

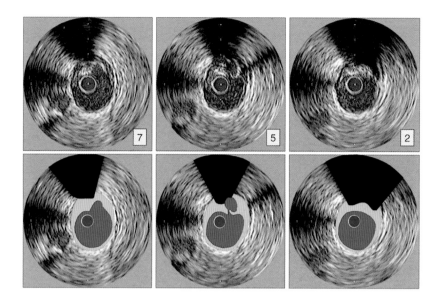

Figure 112 Plaque vulnerability: rupture and calcification (2)
The illustration of the previous figure shows the close relation between the plaque cavity and lesion calcification. However, the pathophysiological relation between rupture, vulnerability and calcification is not well known.

CHAPTERS 5.2.3 AND 7.1, REFERENCES 80, 81

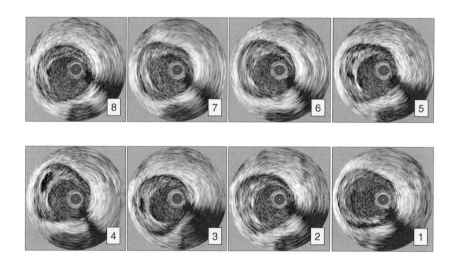

Figure 113 Plaque vulnerability: rupture and intramural hematoma? (1)
In this figure, a plaque ulceration (panels 6 and 7) is continuous with an intramural hematoma (panel 4). While well known in the aorta, the pathophysiology of these entities is less well described in the coronary arteries, and comparative histological studies are not available.

CHAPTER 7.1, REFERENCES 9, 10

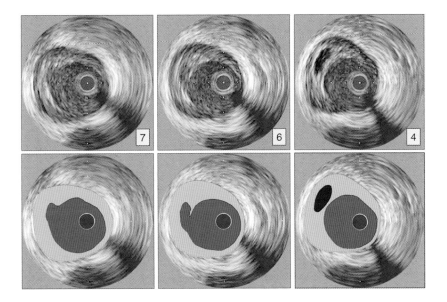

Figure 114 Plaque vulnerability: rupture and intramural hematoma? (2)
This illustration demonstrates the intramural hematoma (no blood flow on video sequence) and the plaque ulceration (blood flow in the cavity).

CHAPTER 7.1, REFERENCES 9, 10

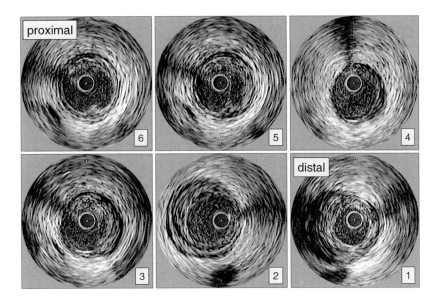

Figure 115 Plaque vulnerability: a multifocal disease process, sequential lesions (1)
Histological studies show that most vulnerable plaques stabilize either without rupture or after episodes of rupture and fibrosis, and only in a few cases do rupture and subsequent thrombosis lead to vessel occlusion and acute coronary syndromes. These studies suggest recurrent episodes of plaque rupture and healing along coronary arteries.

Systemic, e.g. inflammatory, triggers may initiate the multifocal development of vulnerable lesions, increasing the likelihood of an acute clinical event. Therefore the temporal and spatial distributions of vulnerable lesions in the entire coronary tree are highly dynamic and dependent on the clinical situation.

In this figure, six adjacent image slices from a right coronary artery are shown. The patient presented with an acute coronary syndrome with the culprit lesion in the left coronary artery. However, the right coronary artery has ample evidence of vulnerability at several sites including a layered plaque appearance in panel 2 and plaque ulceration in panels 5 and 6.

CHAPTER 7.1, REFERENCES 85, 179–189

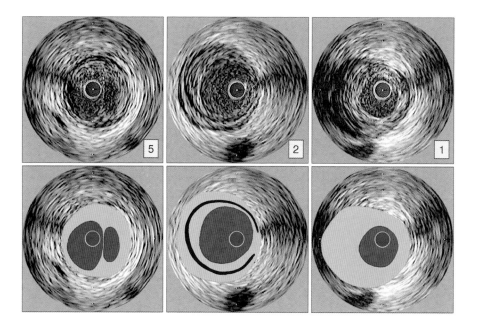

Figure 116 Plaque vulnerability: a diffuse disease process, sequential lesions (2)
The illustration of panels 1, 2, and 5 from the previous figure demonstrates these findings. Panel 1 shows a relatively large eccentric plaque. At site 2, the plaque is layered, suggesting thrombus. Panel 5 shows a plaque rupture.

The examination of sequential lesions in relation to systemic markers of disease activity may help in understanding the influence between local and systemic influences on plaque stability.

CHAPTER 7.1, REFERENCES 85, 179–189

Assessment of plaque burden/volumetric analysis

While the characterization of focal atherosclerotic lesions is important, pathological studies show that coronary artery disease is a systemic process, with a diffuse distribution in the coronary tree. IVUS studies confirm in vivo that plaque distribution is more diffuse than anticipated based on the angiographic appearance of focal stenosis.
Volumetric analysis of atherosclerotic plaque burden is therefore better suited to the assessment of the extent of coronary artery disease.

CHAPTER 7.2, REFERENCES 68, 69, 74, 75, 114, 212

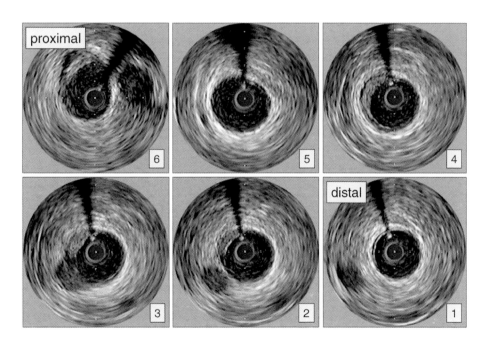

Figure 117 Mild diffuse disease at vessel bifurcation (1)
The assessment of adjacent images slices along coronary segments allows the assessment of the spatial distribution of focal lesions but also the volumetric assessment of the overall plaque burden.

In these consecutive images from a coronary segment, atherosclerotic disease is only found at vessel branches (panels 2, 4 and 6), a site of early atherosclerosis. The overall disease burden is small.

CHAPTER 7.2, REFERENCES 39–44, 68, 69

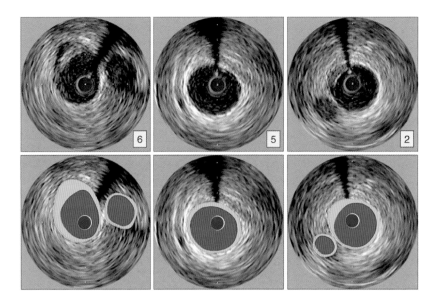

Figure 118 Mild diffuse disease at vessel bifurcation (2)
The mild lesions at sites 2, 5, and 6 of the previous figure are illustrated in this figure. Characteristically, these bifurcation lesions are eccentric with maximal plaque thickness located opposite to the flow divider.

CHAPTER 7.2, REFERENCES 39–44

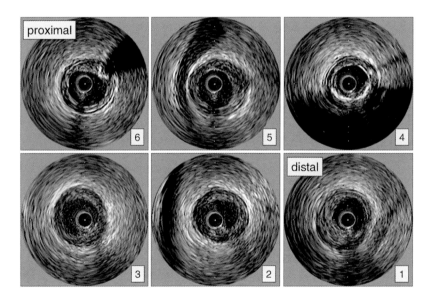

Figure 119 Moderate diffuse disease, morphology (1)
More advanced disease with larger plaque burden is shown in this figure. Adjacent images from a vessel segment demonstrate mild to moderate plaque accumulation in every image, but different morphology. Taken together, these individual plaque areas reflect a moderate plaque burden.

CHAPTER 7.2, REFERENCES 68, 69

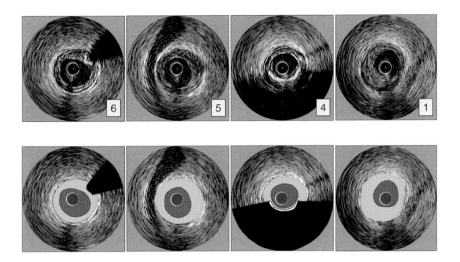

Figure 120 Moderate diffuse disease, morphology (2)
Four images of the previous figure are illustrated here. An eccentric fibrous plaque is found at site 1, and a calcified concentric plaque is found at site 4. The different morphologies in adjacent images demonstrate the heterogeneity of atherosclerotic lesions in the same segment. These observations suggest that local factors may modify the systemic plaque accumulation typical of atherosclerosis.

CHAPTER 7.2, REFERENCES 68, 69

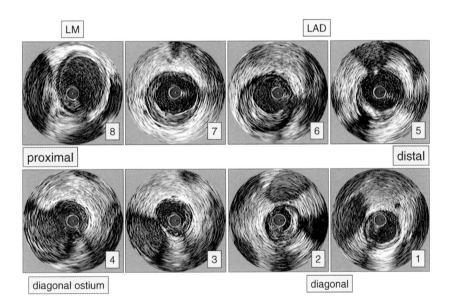

Figure 121 Moderate diffuse disease, plaque burden (1)
Another example of a diffusely diseased vessel segment is shown in these images. Significant plaque accumulation is observed in each image; however, secondary to changes of vessel size, the severity of stenosis is not homogeneous. The plaque area can be measured in each image and added to an overall plaque burden (see Figures 35, 128, 129).

CHAPTER 7.2, REFERENCES 68, 69, 219

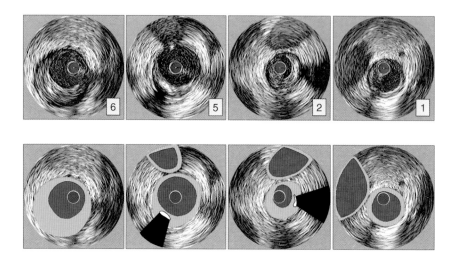

Figure 122 Moderate diffuse disease, plaque burden (2)
Panels 1, 2, 5 and 6 of the previous figure are illustrated. For quantitative volumetric assessment of plaque burden, consecutive plaque area measurements are integrated along a vessel segment (see Figures 35, 128, 129).

The ability of ultrasound to precisely quantify the extent of atherosclerotic plaque is used in regression–progression trials examining serial changes of plaque burden during pharmacological therapy.

CHAPTER 7.2, REFERENCES 68, 69, 219

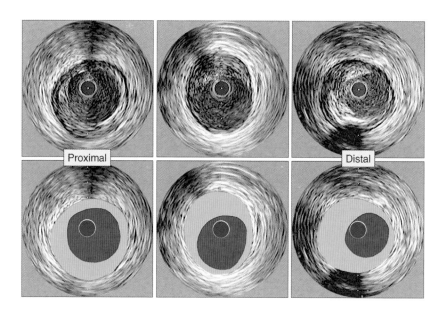

Figure 123 Diffuse disease: lack of reference site
In segments with diffuse disease, it is often difficult to find normal reference sites. In these cases, the lumen, as reflected in the angiogram, may appear almost normal (angiographic mild irregularities) despite large plaque burden.

In this figure, three adjacent images are shown. The size of the lumen tapers from proximal to distal. An angiographic comparison of lumen size would not reveal the relative large plaque burden at all three image slices.

CHAPTER 7.2, REFERENCES 74, 75

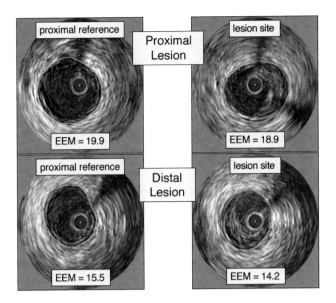

Figure 124 Diffuse disease: sequential lesions (1)

IVUS pullbacks in diffusely diseased vessels often allow the identification of more than one focal lesion. The examination of sequential lesions in relation to systemic markers of disease activity may help to understand the influence between local and systemic influences on plaque morphology.

In this figure, the remodeling responses of two sequential lesions in the same vessel are compared. Both have constrictive remodeling, suggesting the strong influence of systemic factors on remodeling. The remodeling ratios of the proximal and distal lesion are 18.9/19.9 = 0.95 and 14.2/15.5 = 0.92.

CHAPTER 7.2, REFERENCE 216

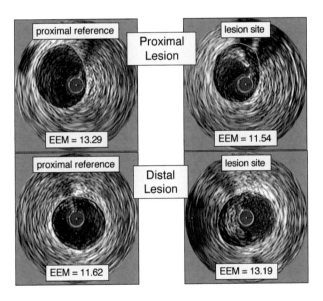

Figure 125 Diffuse disease: sequential lesions (2)

In contrast to figure 124, the remodeling responses of these two sequential lesions in the same coronary segment are discordant. Discordant remodeling response suggests that local factors modify the response of individual lesions, or that lesions in different stages of development are affected in different ways by the systemic environment.

CHAPTER 7.2, REFERENCE 216

Serial examination of progression–regression of coronary artery disease

Serial IVUS examinations of the same lesion or vessel segment can provide important insights into the progression and regression of coronary artery disease and plaque stability.

For the *qualitative* understanding of morphological changes between baseline and follow-up examination, comparison of single matched image slices is very useful.

However, perfect matching is often not possible and the differences between baseline and follow-up images may in part be related to a slightly different image position.

Therefore, volumetric analysis of vessel segments is a preferred alternative for *quantitative* comparisons.

CHAPTER 7.3, REFERENCES 68, 69, 219, 223, 224

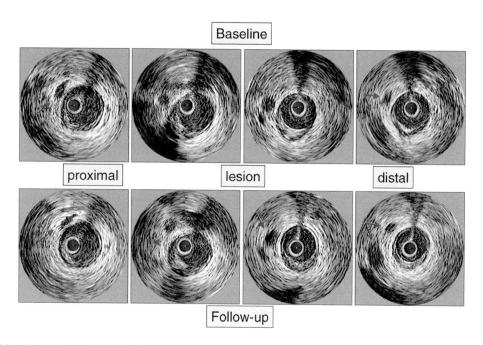

Figure 126 Matched lesions: individual images (1)

Serial studies require matching of the lesion site and comparison of baseline and follow-up images. Individual images are compared side by side, using angiographic and IVUS landmarks (side-branches, pericardium, and cardiac veins) to match sites.

This figure shows images of a mildly stenotic lesion at baseline and follow-up imaging 18 months later. The arterial side-branches (arrows) can serve as landmarks for matching.

CHAPTER 7.3.1, REFERENCES 9, 10, 68, 69, 223, 224

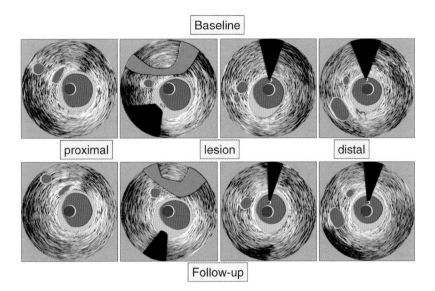

Figure 127 Matched lesions: matching individual images (2)
In this illustration of the previous figure, these landmarks (veins and calcifications) are identified. Matching of individual images at the worst lesion site is limited by changes in plaque size and morphology between baseline and follow-up.

CHAPTER 7.3.1, REFERENCES 9, 10, 68, 69, 223, 224

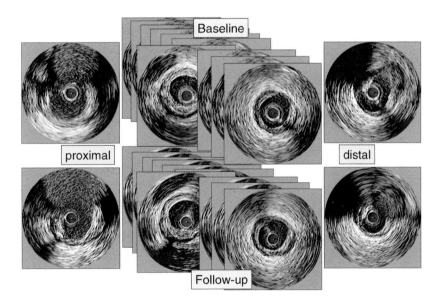

Figure 128 Matched lesions: matching segments (1)
For serial, volumetric analysis, a vessel segment is selected between two fiduciary points (Chapter 4.8). The ultrasound catheter is placed beyond the distal fiduciary point and a motorized pullback is performed through the selected segment. Multiple, evenly spaced image slices (selected at 0.5–1 mm intervals or based on ECG gating) are obtained and analyzed. In this and the next figure, the volumetric approach is illustrated. Images of the fiduciary points and several image slices in the selected segment are shown.

CHAPTER 7.3.1, REFERENCES 9, 10, 68, 69, 219

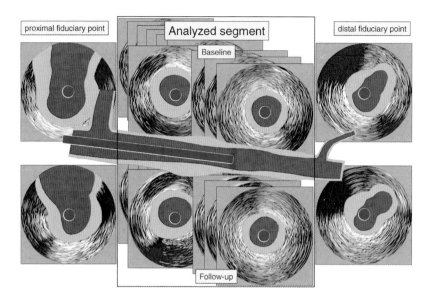

Figure 129 Matched lesions: matching segments (2)
This figure is an illustration of the volumetric assessment of plaque burden. Studies show that plaque plus media volume calculated in this manner is highly reproducible and that serial studies can detect very small changes in atheroma volume.

CHAPTER 7.3.1, REFERENCES 9, 10, 68, 69, 219

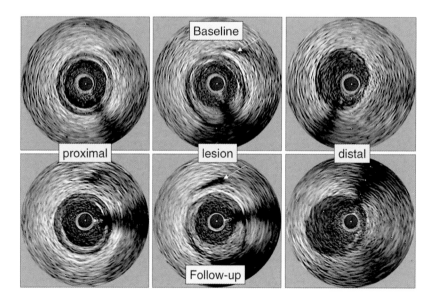

Figure 130 Matched lesions: location (1)
This figure shows images of a lesion site and adjacent reference sites at baseline and follow-up imaging 18 months later. The eccentric plaque and the venous branch on the opposite site (arrow) allow a relative reliable match.

CHAPTER 7.3.1, REFERENCES 9, 10, 68, 69, 220, 223, 224

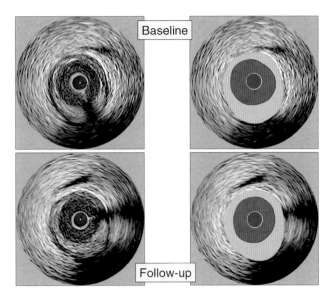

Figure 131 Matched lesions: location (2)
In this illustration of the previous figure, only the lesion site is shown at baseline and follow-up imaging. The plaque area is almost unchanged in size and morphology.

CHAPTER 7.3.1, REFERENCES 9, 10, 68, 69, 220, 223, 224

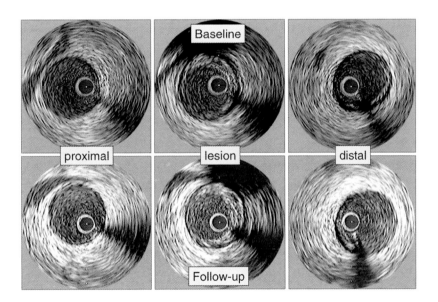

Figure 132 Matched lesions: limitations – image rotation (1)
This figure shows matched images of a lesion site and adjacent reference sites at baseline and follow-up imaging 18 months later. The venous branch serves as landmark.

In comparison to the baseline image, the image at follow-up is rotated clockwise by about 20°. Rotation can make the visual process of matching more difficult.

CHAPTER 7.3.1, REFERENCES 9, 10, 68, 69

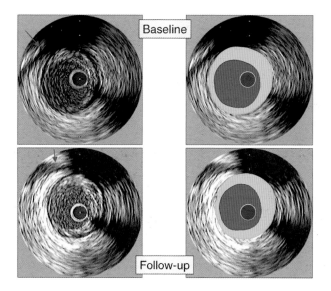

Figure 133 Matched lesions: limitations – image rotation (2)

This illustration of the previous figure shows the lesion site at baseline and follow-up.

The differences in rotation can be observed by the different positions of the venous structure (arrow). The lesion is almost unchanged in size but appears more echogenic in the images at follow-up. However, a comparison of the surrounding connective tissue demonstrates that the entire image is brighter and that plaque and adventitia have similar echodensities. The apparent difference in plaque echogenicity is caused by different image settings.

CHAPTER 7.3.1, REFERENCES 9, 10, 68, 69

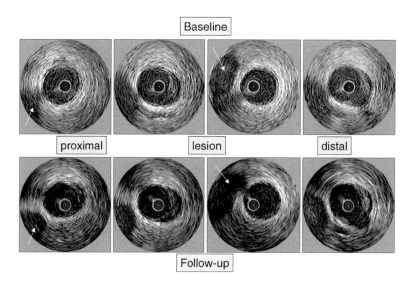

Figure 134 Matched lesions: limitation – system settings (1)

This figure shows adjacent images of a lesion at baseline and follow-up imaging 18 months later. The arterial side-branches (arrows) can serve as landmarks for matching.

Differences in system settings at baseline and follow-up are obvious. The overall gain was lower in the follow-up images, giving the plaque a more echolucent appearance. It is important to observe these differences in order to avoid misinterpretation of morphology in serial studies.

CHAPTER 7.3.1, REFERENCES 9, 10, 68, 69

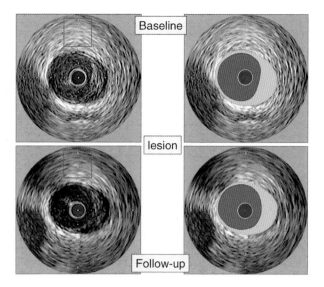

Figure 135 Matched lesions: limitation – system settings (2)
The illustration of the previous figure demonstrates the differences in image setting.
The more echolucent appearance of the lesion at follow-up is secondary to a lower image gain at follow-up. This becomes obvious by comparing the echogenicities of the adventitia (small squares in left panels).

CHAPTER 7.3.1, REFERENCES 9, 10, 68, 69

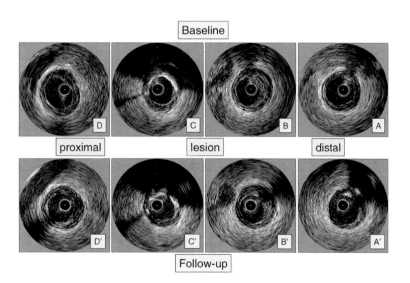

Figure 136 Matched lesions: morphology (1)
This figure shows matched images of several adjacent sites of a coronary segment at baseline and follow-up imaging 18 months later.
Plaque morphologies are different in adjacent images, with notable calcifications in panels A and C. Serial imaging allows the observation of morphological changes over time.
In a recent serial IVUS study, examining 131 patients at baseline and after 12 months' treatment with lipid-lowering medications, echogenicity increased to a larger extent in the treatment group than in the control group, suggesting a possible relationship between lesion stability and morphology.

CHAPTER 7.3.1, REFERENCES 68, 69, 219

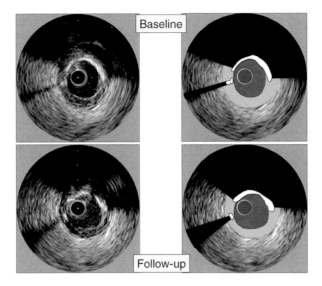

Figure 137 Matched lesions: morphology (2)
The illustration of the baseline and follow-up images at site C of the previous figure show the similarity in the arterial wall calcification in this artery.
The serial examination of lesions will further clarify the role of coronary calcifications in plaque stability/vulnerability (see Chapter 5.2.3).

CHAPTER 7.3.1, REFERENCES 68, 69, 80, 81, 219, 220, 223

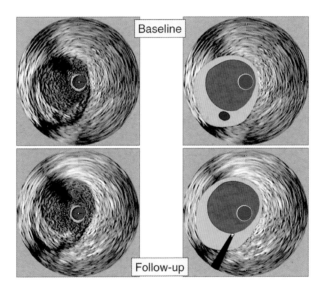

Figure 138 Matched lesions: morphology – echolucent core (1)
The serial observation of lesions with characteristics of vulnerability will be of particular interest. In this figure, an example of a plaque with heterogeneous morphology is shown at baseline and follow-up. A small echolucent core is demonstrated at baseline (7 o'clock position). The echolucent core appears smaller with more calcification at follow-up. It is an attractive hypothesis that this finding reflects changes of a necrotic core. However, the significance of these findings is currently unclear.

CHAPTER 7.3.1, REFERENCES 68, 69, 80, 81, 203, 204, 219, 223

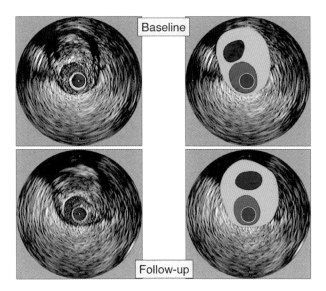

Figure 139 Matched lesions: morphology – echolucent core (2)

In this figure, another example of a heterogeneous plaque with an echolucent core is shown at baseline and follow-up. Such lesions are thought to represent unstable lesion (see Chapter 5.2.8).

Surprisingly, in this example, plaque morphology, including the central echolucent area, is very similar at follow-up 18 months later.

CHAPTER 7.3.1, REFERENCES 68, 69, 204, 219

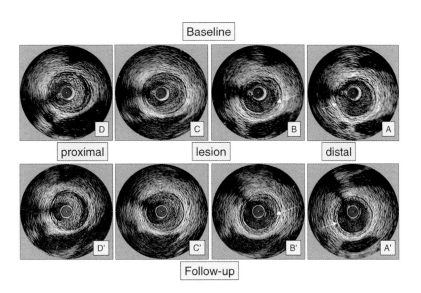

Figure 140 Matched lesions: thrombus? (1)

In this example, matched baseline and 1-month follow-up images are shown of a coronary segment containing a lesion with characteristics suggestive of thrombus. Panels D and D' (the most proximal site) show a echodense lesion. In panels C and C', the plaque has both echodense and echolucent components, a finding consistent with layers of thrombus. In panels A and B, a focal area of echolucency is seen at baseline (arrow).

CHAPTER 7.3.1, REFERENCES 68, 69, 82

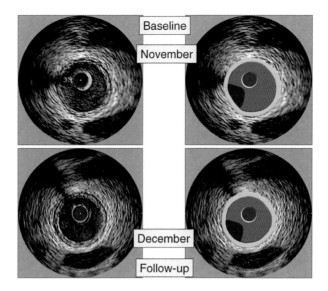

Figure 141 Matched lesions: thrombus (2)
The illustration of panel A from Figure 140, shows that this focal echolucent filling defect is still present at 1-month follow-up, suggesting either thrombus or a very echolucent plaque.

CHAPTER 7.3.1, REFERENCES 68, 69, 82

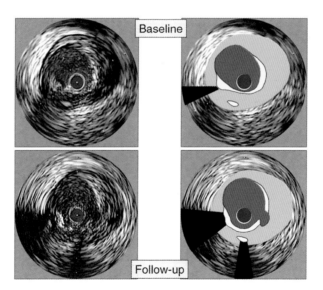

Figure 142 Matched lesions: rupture at follow-up (1)
Recent IVUS studies have demonstrated plaque ulceration and rupture at non-culprit lesion sites. An exciting aspect of serial imaging will be the longitudinal observation of such lesions with characteristics of instability and rupture.
In this example, matched lesion sites are shown at baseline and follow-up after 18 months. The lesion site at follow-up shows evidence of rupture at the 5 o'clock position. The description of plaque morphology at baseline may eventually allow the finding of characteristics of plaques at risk to rupture.

CHAPTER 7.3.1, REFERENCES 68, 69, 85–87, 179–189

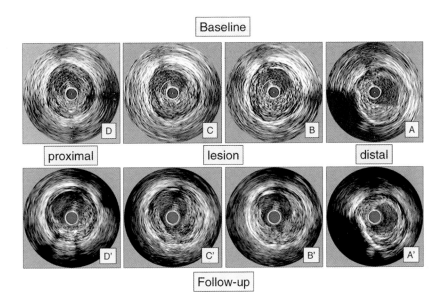

Figure 143 Matched lesions: rupture at follow-up (2)
Another example of plaque rupture at the follow-up examination is shown in this and the next two figures. Matched lesion sites are shown at baseline and follow-up. Sites B and C show evidence of rupture at follow-up.

CHAPTER 7.3.1, REFERENCES 68, 69, 85–87, 179–189

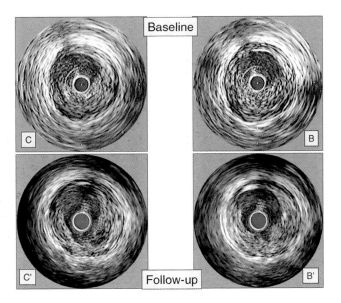

Figure 144 Matched lesions: rupture at follow-up (2)
This figure shows enlarged images of sites B and C of the previous figure. The plaque cavity at follow-up is obvious at the 5 o'clock position.

CHAPTER 7.3.1, REFERENCES 85–87, 179–189

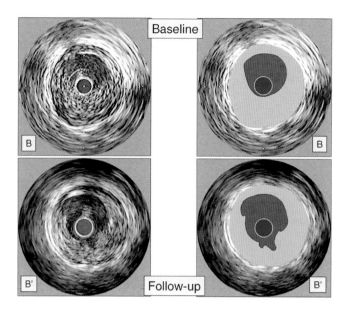

Figure 145 Matched lesions: rupture at follow-up (3)
This figure illustrates the findings of site B from the previous figure. The shallow plaque cavity (6 o'clock position) is demonstrated.

CHAPTER 7.3.1, REFERENCES 85–87, 179–189

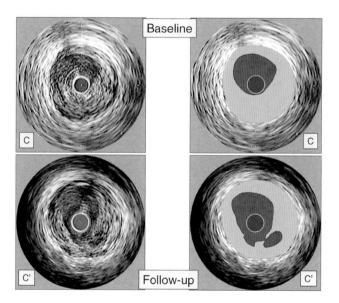

Figure 146 Matched lesions: rupture at follow-up (4)
This figure illustrates the findings of site C from Figure 144. The cavity is deeper than at site B (Figure 145) and is partially separated from the lumen by an echodense structure, which likely reflects the fibrous cap.

CHAPTER 7.3.1, REFERENCES 85–87, 179–189

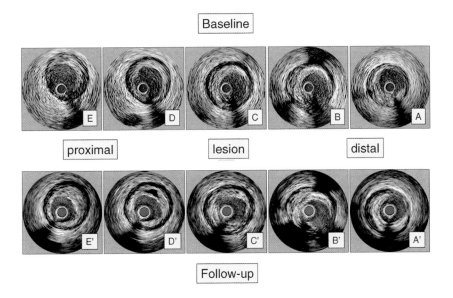

Figure 147 Matched lesions: rupture and intramural hematoma (1)
An example of plaque rupture at the follow-up examination associated with a suspected intramural hematoma is shown in this and the next two figures. Matched lesion sites are shown at baseline and follow-up. Sites C and D show evidence of intramural hematoma and rupture at follow-up, respectively. (see Figure 98)

CHAPTER 7.3.1, REFERENCES 179–189

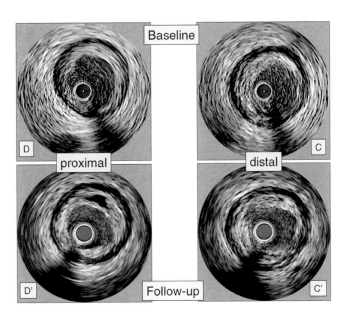

Figure 148 Matched lesions: rupture and intramural hematoma (2)
This figure shows enlarged images of sites C and D of the previous figure.

The echolucent area in image D' probably represents an intramural thrombus. Image C' demonstrates evidence of plaque rupture at the 10 o'clock position.

CHAPTER 7.3.1, REFERENCES 179–189

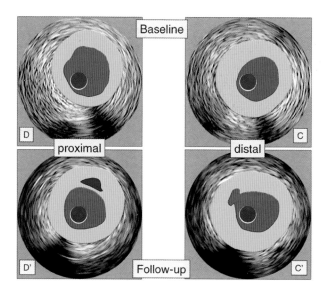

Figure 149 Matched lesions: rupture and intramural hematoma (3)

This figure shows illustrations of images of sites C and D of the previous figure.

The echolucent area in image D' probably represents a thrombus/intramural hematoma. Image C' demonstrates evidence of plaque rupture at the 10 o'clock position.

CHAPTER 7.3.1, REFERENCES 179–189

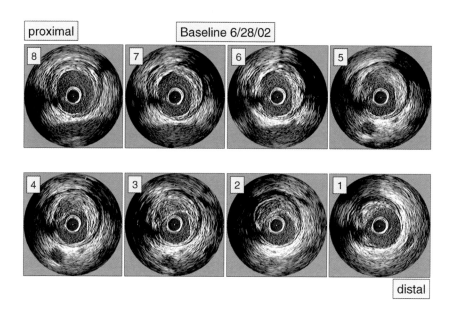

Figure 150 Matched lesions: rupture at baseline (1)

In this figure, a plaque with evidence of rupture at baseline is shown. The findings are explained and illustrated in the following figure.

CHAPTER 7.3.1, REFERENCES 85–87, 179–189

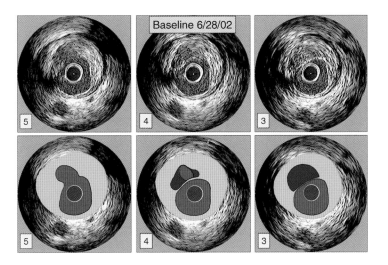

Figure 151 Matched lesions: rupture at baseline (2)
The illustrations of panels 3, 4, and 5 of the previous figure show the structures of the plaque in detail.

The thin echodense structure in panel 3, separating lumen and plaque, may represent a fibrous cap. In more proximal images (panels 4 and 5), this structure is interrupted with flow in the cavity, suggesting plaque rupture.

CHAPTER 7.3.1, REFERENCES 85–87, 179–189

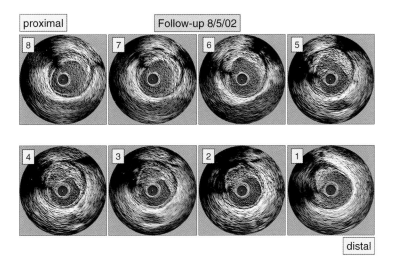

Figure 152 Matched lesions: rupture at baseline (3)
In this figure, the same vessel segment seen in the previous figures is shown at follow-up 1 month later.

The slice position of the eight images has been matched carefully to those in Figure 150. The similarity of plaque morphology is striking and is illustrated in the next two figures.

CHAPTER 7.3.1, REFERENCES 85–87, 179–189

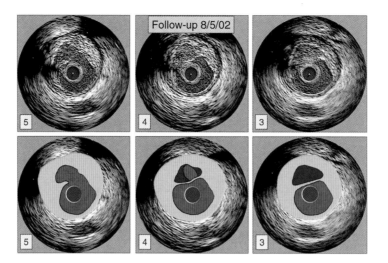

Figure 153 Matched lesions: rupture at baseline (4)

The illustrations of panels 3, 4, and 5 of the previous figure show the structures of the plaque in detail.

Again seen is the thin echodense structure in panel 3 which may represent a fibrous cap. In more proximal images (panels 4 and 5), this structure is interrupted with flow in the cavity, suggesting plaque rupture (compare to baseline, Figure 151).

CHAPTER 7.3.1, REFERENCES 85–87, 179–189

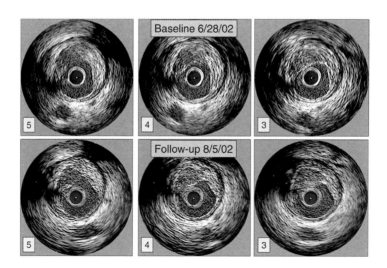

Figure 154 Matched lesions: rupture at baseline (5)

The comparison between baseline and follow-up shows almost no morphological changes.

This example demonstrates how serial observation of lesion morphology could improve our understanding of lesion progression–regression. A limitation of anatomic observations is that biochemical and ultrastructural changes associated with lesion progression, regression, and vulnerability are probably not reflected in morphology. The results from imaging studies, therefore, need to be compared to markers of systemic disease activity (e.g. inflammatory serum markers).

CHAPTER 7.3.1, REFERENCES 85–87, 179–189

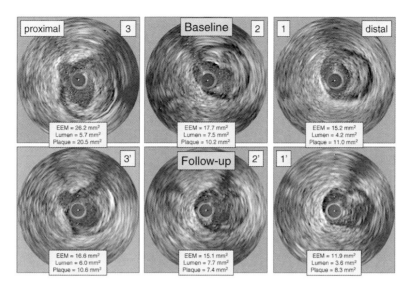

Figure 155 Matched lesions: plaque rupture and remodeling (1)
In this figure a lesion site with evidence of plaque rupture at baseline and follow-up and adjacent sites are shown. At follow-up, the lesion site and reference sites show decrease in vessel size (constrictive remodeling) but also a decrease in plaque size.

In recent investigations, plaque rupture has been described as initiating a form of 'healing' process, characterized by fibrosis, which could be related to the constrictive remodeling response.

CHAPTER 7.3.1, REFERENCES 68, 69,85–87, 179–188

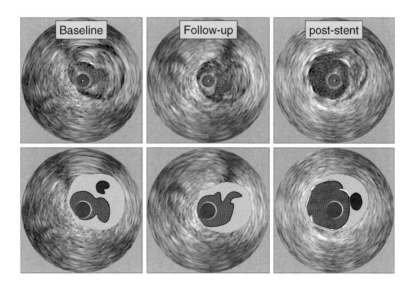

Figure 156 Matched lesions: plaque rupture and remodeling (2)
The illustrations demonstrate the morphologic findings at the lesion site at baseline and follow-up. At follow-up, the patient underwent stenting of the lesion site (right panels).

CHAPTER 7.3.1, REFERENCES 68, 69, 85–87, 179–188

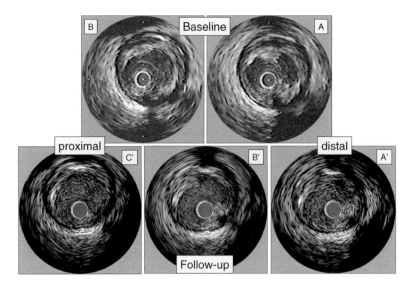

Figure 157 Matched lesions: rupture and vessel wall cavity (1)
The careful examination of non-culprit vessel segments occasionally shows larger cavities in the vessel wall, which could be chronic sequelae after plaque rupture. However, the significance of such findings is currently unclear.

In this figure, such a cavity is shown at baseline and follow-up imaging 18 months later.

CHAPTER 7.3.1, REFERENCES 85–86, 179–180

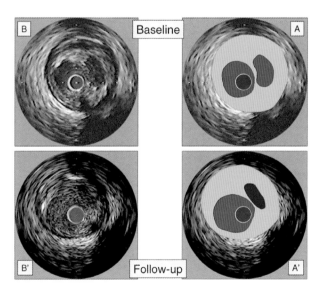

Figure 158 Matched lesions: rupture and vessel wall cavity (2)
The illustrations of sites A and B from the previous figure demonstrate the findings at baseline and follow-up.

Site A shows a cavity in the vessel wall which is separated from the lumen by a echodense structure. In the video sequences, blood flow could be seen at baseline but not at follow-up suggesting interval thrombosis.

Site B shows a larger cavity, which is in direct contact with the lumen, and is unchanged during follow-up.

CHAPTER 7.3.1, REFERENCES 85–87, 179–189

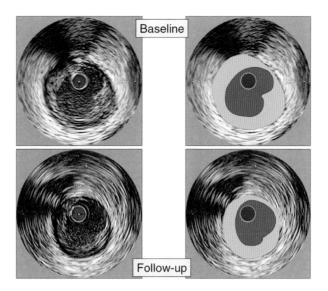

Figure 159 Matched lesions: vessel wall cavity – remnant of rupture?
In this figure, another example of a vessel wall cavity is shown at baseline and follow-up imaging 18 months later. There is no significant morphological change.

It is important to mention that a joining side-branch can have a similar appearance and therefore a careful review of adjacent images is important (Figure 65)

CHAPTER 7.3.1, REFERENCES 85–87, 179–189

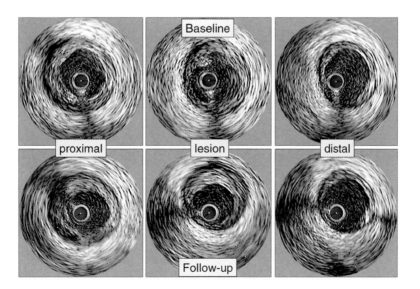

Figure 160 Matched lesions: healed rupture (1)
In this example matched lesion sites are shown at baseline and follow-up. The lesion site at baseline (middle panel, 12 o'clock) shows evidence of rupture. In contrast to the previous figures, there is change during follow-up. The vessel wall cavity appears to be filled by echodense material at follow-up.

CHAPTER 7.3.1, REFERENCES 68, 69, 85–87, 179–189, 203, 204

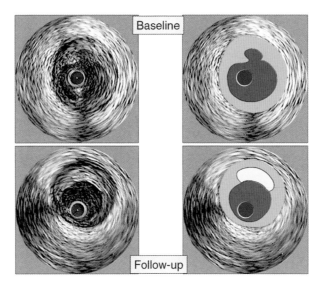

Figure 161 Matched lesions: healed rupture (2)
At follow-up, the rupture is not evident and no cavity is found. The corresponding area of the lesion appears echodense. The EEM area at follow-up is smaller, suggesting constrictive (negative) remodeling.

Recent histological studies suggest that plaque rupture and healing are frequent events, which are most often asymptomatic. It is unclear if the finding in this figure corresponds to such a 'healed lesion'.

CHAPTER 7.3.1, REFERENCES 68, 69, 85–87, 179–189, 203, 204

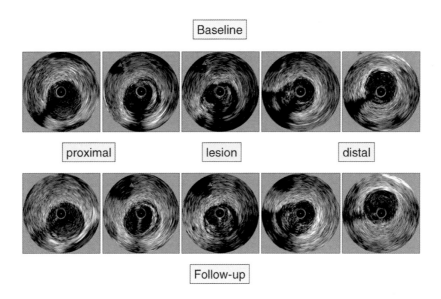

Figure 162 Matched lesions: severity – no change (1)
An exciting application of serial IVUS imaging is the observation of changes in plaque burden. The progression of plaque burden has been examined in a small studies comparing matched lesion sites of moderate lesions at baseline and follow-up.

This figure shows five adjacent images of a coronary segment at baseline and follow-up imaging 18 months later. The arterial side-branch (arrow) can serve as landmark.

CHAPTER 7.3.2, REFERENCES 68, 69, 219, 220, 223, 224

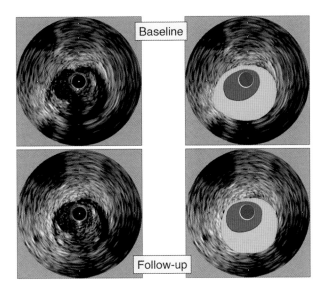

Figure 163 Matched lesions: severity – no change (2)
In this illustration of Figure 162, the lesion site is shown at baseline and follow-up.

The lesion is almost unchanged and can be readily recognized by its eccentricity and location relative to the arterial side-branch.

The similarity of the lesions in serial examinations is often striking. Serial observation of lesions will eventually clarify to what extent changes in plaque composition are reflected in imaging studies.

CHAPTER 7.3.2, REFERENCES 68, 69, 219, 220, 223, 224

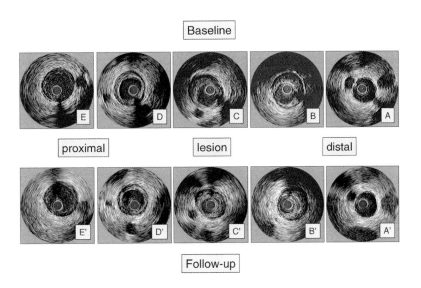

Figure 164 Matched lesions: severity – progression (1.1)
This figure shows images of several adjacent sites of a coronary segment at baseline and follow-up imaging 18 months later.

The arterial side-branches serve as landmarks.

The lesion site (panels B and C) clearly shows a significant increase in plaque burden between baseline and follow-up.

CHAPTER 7.3.2, REFERENCES 68, 69, 219, 220, 223, 224

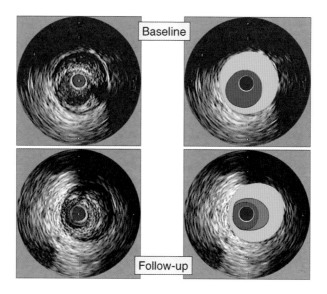

Figure 165 Matched lesions: severity – progression (1.2)

The illustration of the lesion site (panel B from the previous image) clearly shows an increase in plaque burden with a smaller lumen at follow-up.

The layered appearance with different echogenicity of the new tissue reminds one of in-stent restenosis (Figure 34).

Recent histological studies describe repeated episodes of plaque rupture as a common event in plaque progression. This is associated with a layered plaque morphology. However, it is unclear if the morphological changes observed in this figure correlate to specific histological changes.

CHAPTER 7.3.2, REFERENCES 68, 69, 219, 220, 223, 224

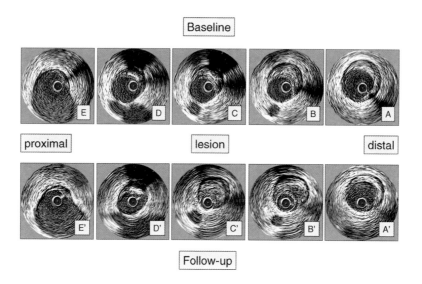

Figure 166 Matched lesions: severity – progression (2.1)

This figure shows another example of significant progression at the lesion site. Images of several adjacent sites of a coronary segment at baseline and follow-up imaging 18 months later are shown.

The lesion site (panels B and C) clearly shows progressive plaque burden.

CHAPTER 7.3.2, REFERENCES 68, 69, 219, 220, 223, 224

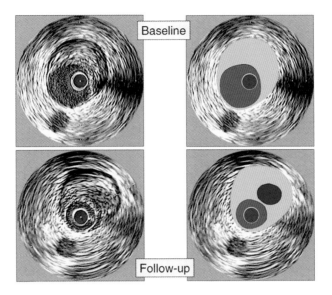

Figure 167 Matched lesions: severity – progression (2.2)
The illustration of the lesion site (panel B from the previous image) clearly shows an increase in plaque burden and a smaller lumen at follow-up.

At follow-up, the plaque has a heterogeneous appearance with an echolucent core, which could represent a necrotic core.

CHAPTER 7.3.2, REFERENCES 68, 69, 219, 220, 223, 224

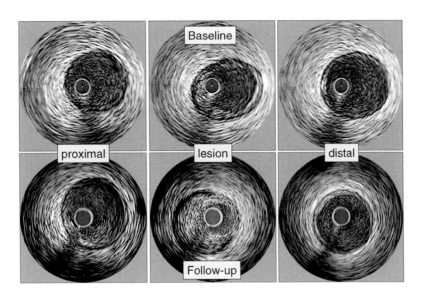

Figure 168 Matched lesions: severity – progression (3.1)
Another example of plaque progression is shown in this figure. The increased plaque area and decreased lumen area of the lesion site at follow-up are obvious.

CHAPTER 7.3.2, REFERENCES 68, 69, 219, 220, 223, 224

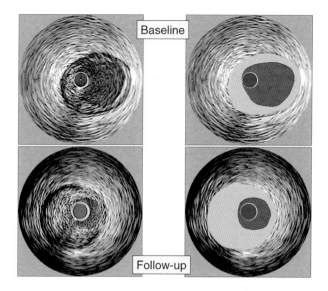

Figure 169 Matched lesions: severity – progression (3.2)
The illustration of the lesion site clearly shows an increase in plaque burden with a smaller lumen at follow-up.

CHAPTER 7.3.2, REFERENCES 68, 69, 219, 220, 223, 224

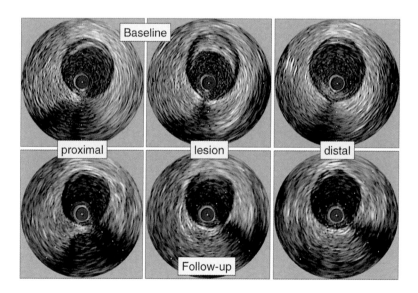

Figure 170 Matched lesions: severity – regression (1.1)
It is likely that plaque stabilization, e.g. during pharmacological treatment, is associated with plaque regression. Previous small serial studies examining plaque burden during lipid-lowering therapy demonstrated an attenuated plaque growth in the treatment group.

This figure shows matched images of a lesion site at baseline and follow-up imaging 18 months later. The plaque area at the lesion site appears smaller at follow-up, suggesting plaque regression.

CHAPTER 7.3.2, REFERENCES 68, 69, 203, 204, 219, 220, 223, 224

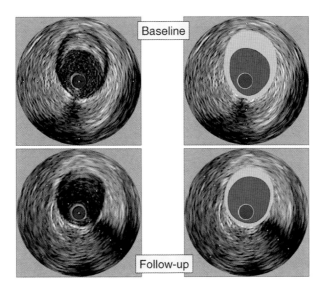

Figure 171 Matched lesions: severity – regression (1.2)
The illustration of the lesion site demonstrates the decrease in plaque area.

Although matching has been performed very carefully and adjacent images were included in the analysis, the matching of single images has limitations, because slight differences in image location may result in false-positive findings. This limitation is the rationale for volumetric IVUS analysis.

CHAPTER 7.3.2, REFERENCES 68, 69, 203, 204, 219, 220, 223, 224

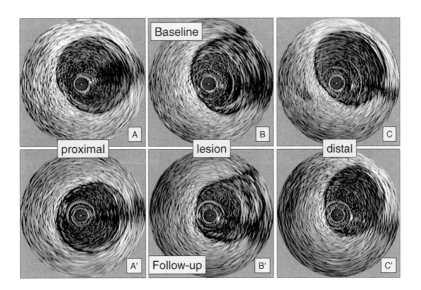

Figure 172 Matched lesions: severity – regression (2.1)
In this figure, another example of lesion regression is shown. Plaque size, but also EEM area, is decreased at follow-up.

CHAPTER 7.3.2, REFERENCES 68, 69, 203, 204, 219, 220, 223, 224

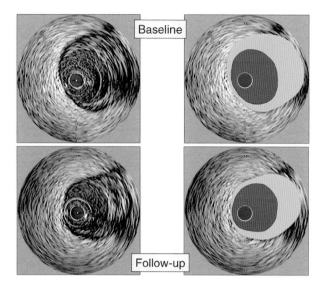

Figure 173 Matched lesions: severity – regression (2.2)

The illustration of the lesion site from the previous figures demonstrates the decrease in plaque and EEM size. It is an attractive hypothesis that plaque regression may be associated with negative remodeling.

CHAPTER 7.3.2, REFERENCES 68, 69, 203, 204, 219, 220, 223, 224

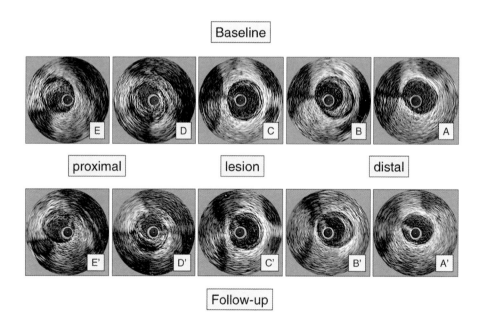

Figure 174 Matched lesions: severity – regression (3.1)

Another example of possible plaque regression is shown in this figure. Again, matched images of several adjacent sites of a coronary segment at baseline and follow-up imaging 18 months later are shown.

The plaque areas at several sites (B and E) appears smaller at follow-up, suggesting plaque regression. However, the most severe lesion (site D) appears relatively stable. Serial volumetric analysis of plaque burden will provide invaluable insight into plaque progression and regression.

CHAPTER 7.3.2, REFERENCES 68, 69, 203, 204, 219, 220, 223, 224

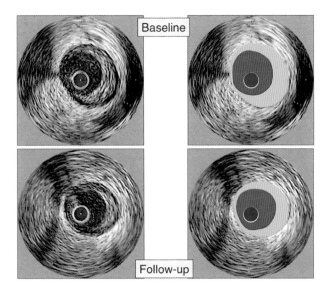

Figure 175 Matched lesions: severity – regression (3.2)
This illustration of site B from the previous figure demonstrates the decrease in plaque area.

CHAPTER 7.3.2, REFERENCES 68, 69, 203, 204, 219, 220, 223, 224

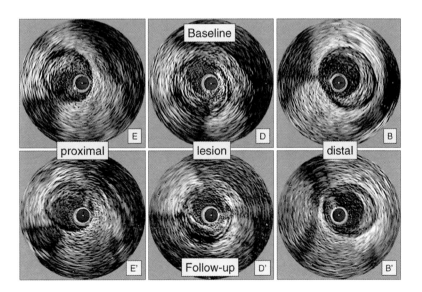

Figure 176 Matched lesions: severity – regression (3.3)
These images compare sites E, D, and B from Figure 174 at baseline and follow-up. The plaque areas at sites B and E appear smaller at follow-up, suggesting plaque regression. The most severe site (D) appears relatively stable. The independent progression/ regression of adjacent lesions suggests that both focal and systemic factors influence individual lesions.

CHAPTER 7.3.2, REFERENCES 68, 69, 203, 204, 219, 220, 223, 224

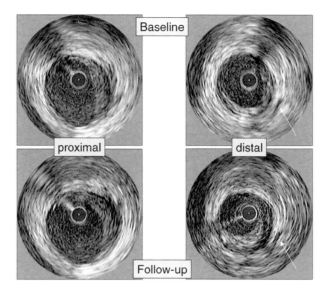

Figure 177 Serial IVUS: sequential lesions (1.1)

In long pullbacks through coronary arteries, it is common to find more than one focal lesion in adjacent segments. The serial observation of such sequential lesions or lesions in different arteries will allow the differentiation of whether the factors causing progression/regression, remodeling, and vulnerability are focal or systemic.

In this figure, two sequential lesions from the same artery are shown.

CHAPTER 7.2.1, REFERENCES 68, 69, 216

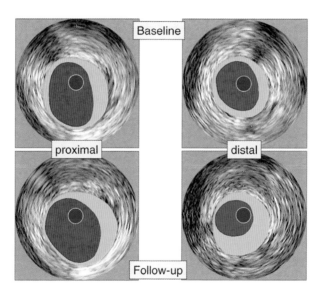

Figure 178 Serial IVUS: sequential lesions (1.2)

The illustration of the two lesions show that plaque progression in the distal lesion is associated with luminal compromise.

However, the small increase in plaque burden in the proximal lesion is accommodated by positive remodeling. It is an attractive hypothesis that both plaque growth and remodeling response may by affected by focal and systemic factors.

CHAPTER 7.2.1, REFERENCES 68, 69, 216

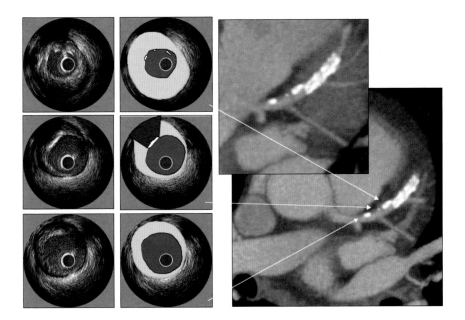

Figure 179 Comparison between IVUS and coronary computed tomography
The non-invasive assessment of coronary plaque morphology and plaque burden is an exciting area of current research with computed tomography and magnetic resonance imaging.

This image illustrates the comparison between IVUS and multidetector computed tomography (MDCT). A complex plaque with calcified and non-calcified components is seen in the LAD proximal to the stented mid-LAD segment.

CHAPTERS 1.3.6 AND 8, REFERENCES 29–31,214, 215, 224–226

Case study 1
Lesion progression and subsequent PCI

Figures 180–182 show images of a LAD artery segment at baseline and follow-up imaging 18 months later. Because of disease progression, PCI was performed at follow-up.

CHAPTER 7.3.2, REFERENCES 68, 69

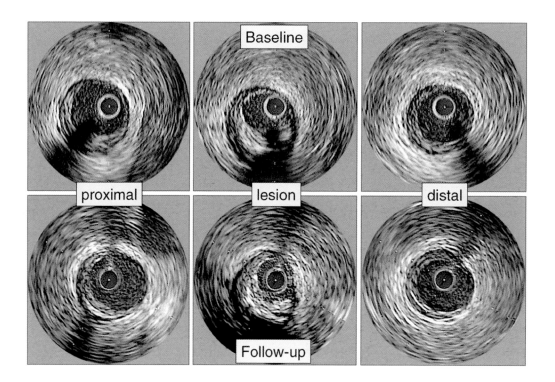

Figure 180 Case study: progression (1.1)
This figure shows matched images of the lesion and reference sites in the LAD at baseline and follow-up imaging 18 months later.

The patient was symptomatic with unstable angina pectoris at follow-up.

CHAPTER 7.3.2, REFERENCES 68, 69

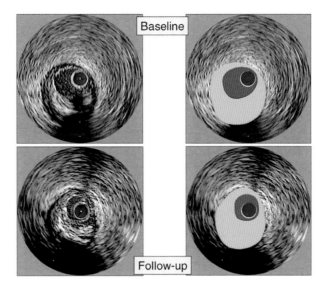

Figure 181 Case study: progression (1.2)
The illustration of the lesion site demonstrates the significant increase in plaque area and the tight luminal stenosis at follow-up. The lesion calcifications in the 6 o'clock position are similar at baseline and follow-up.

CHAPTER 7.3.2, REFERENCES 68, 69

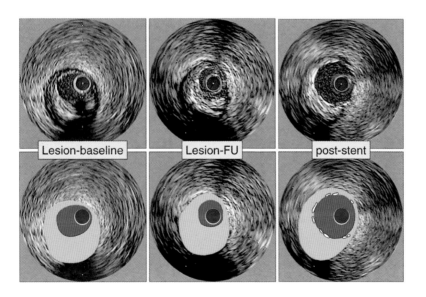

Figure 182 Case study: progression (1.4)
Based on the patient's symptoms and these morphological findings, PCI was performed.
    Matched images of the lesion site at baseline, follow-up, and after intervention are shown.

CHAPTER 7.3.2, REFERENCES 68, 69

Case study 2
PCI of lesion site and regression of an additional lesion

Figures 183–190 show angiographic and intravascular ultrasound images of a severe LAD stenosis at baseline and follow-up. The patient underwent PCI of the LAD. IVUS was performed in the LCX at baseline and follow-up imaging 18 months later as part of a study protocol observing plaque burden during lipid-lowering therapy. At follow-up there is angiographic restenosis inside the LAD stent. However, IVUS of the LCX segment shows regression of plaque burden.

CHAPTER 7.3.2, REFERENCES 68, 69, 219, 223, 224

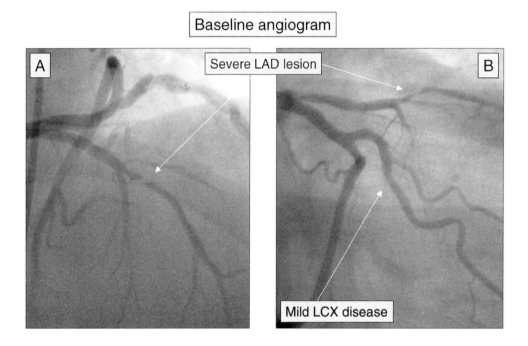

Figure 183 Case study: regression (2.1)
The angiogram at baseline shows a severe LAD lesion and mild disease in a lateral branch of the LCX. However the main LCX has only minimal luminal irregularities.

CHAPTER 7.3.2, REFERENCES 68, 69, 219, 223, 224

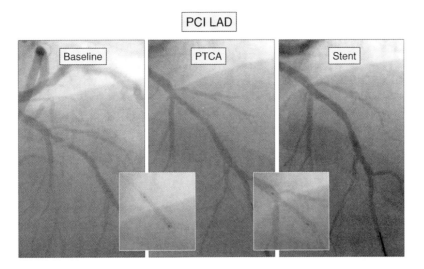

Figure 184 Case study: regression (2.2)
PCI of the LAD was performed. In this figure, pre- and post-interventional angiographic images are shown.

CHAPTER 7.3.2, REFERENCES 68, 69, 219, 223, 224

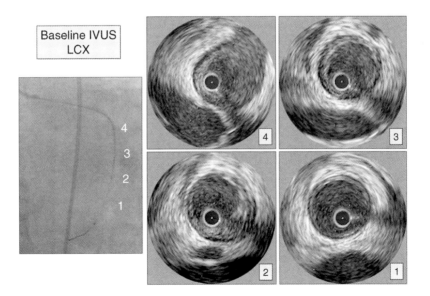

Figure 185 Case study: regression (2.3)
IVUS was performed in the angiographically normal main LCX as part of a study protocol. The panel on the left shows the
  IVUS catheter in the LCX (compare to panel B, Figure 182). The IVUS images on the right show images of several adjacent sites of the LCX at baseline. There is an eccentric atherosclerotic lesion at site 2.

CHAPTER 7.3.2, REFERENCES 68, 69, 219, 223, 224

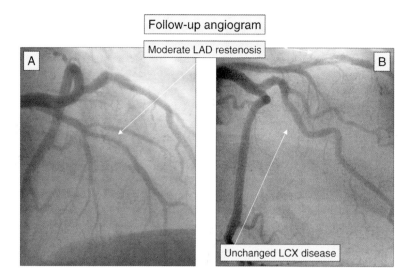

Figure 186 Case study: regression (2.4)

The angiogram at follow-up shows moderate in-stent restenosis at the LAD lesion. The angiographic appearance of the LCX is unchanged (compare to figure 182)

CHAPTER 7.3.2, REFERENCES 68, 69, 219, 223, 224

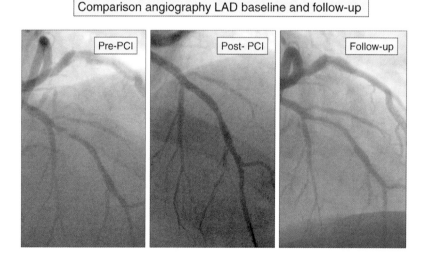

Figure 187 Case study: regression (2.5)

In this figure the comparisons of the angiogram at baseline (pre- and post-intervention) and follow-up are shown, demonstrating the development of in-stent restenosis.

CHAPTER 7.3.2, REFERENCES 68, 69, 219, 223, 224

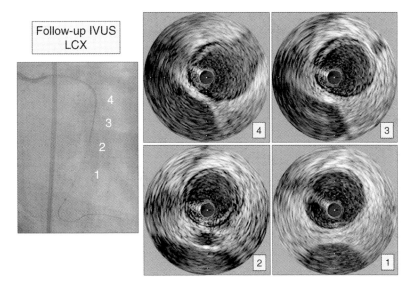

Figure 188 Case study: regression (2.6)
Repeat IVUS was performed in the LCX as part of a study protocol at follow-up during lipid-lowering therapy. Similar to Figure 184 the panel on the left shows the IVUS catheter in the LCX (compare to Figure 185, panel B). The IVUS images on the right show images of several adjacent sites of the LCX at baseline.

There is an eccentric lesion at site 2, but the plaque burden is reduced in comparison to the baseline images (Figure 184).

CHAPTER 7.3.2, REFERENCES 68, 69, 217, 223, 224

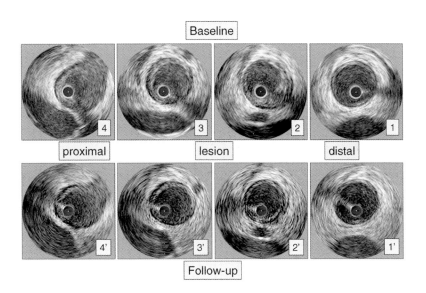

Figure 189 Case study: regression (2.7)
In this figure, matched IVUS images of the angiographic mild LCX lesion site at baseline and follow-up are shown, demonstrating regression of the LCX lesion.

CHAPTER 7.3.2, REFERENCES 68, 69, 219, 223, 22

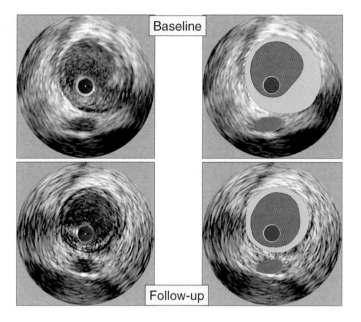

Figure 190 Case study: regression (2.8)
The illustration of the lesion site (panel 2 of previous image) at baseline and follow-up demonstrates the reduced plaque burden at follow-up.

CHAPTER 7.3.2, REFERENCES 68, 69, 219, 223, 224

References

1. Nissen SE, Yock P. Intravascular ultrasound: novel pathophysiological insights and current clinical applications. *Circulation* 2001;103:604–16

2. Yock PG, Linker DT, Angelsen BA. Two-dimensional intravascular ultrasound: technical development and initial clinical experience. *J Am Soc Echocardiogr* 1989;2:296–304

3. Hodgson JM, Graham SP, Savakus AD, *et al.* Clinical percutaneous imaging of coronary anatomy using an over-the-wire ultrasound catheter system. *Int J Card Imaging* 1989;4:187–93

4. Nissen SE, Grines CL, Gurley JC, *et al.* Application of a new phased-array ultrasound imaging catheter in the assessment of vascular dimensions: in vivo comparison to cineangiography. *Circulation* 1990;81:660–6

5. Tobis JM, Mallery J, Mahon D, *et al.* Intravascular ultrasound imaging of human coronary arteries *in vivo*: analysis of tissue characterizations with comparison to *in vitro* histological specimens. *Circulation* 1991;83:913–26

6. Maheswaran B, Leung CY, Gutfinger DE, *et al.* Intravascular ultrasound appearance of normal and mildly diseased coronary arteries: correlation with histologic specimens. *Am Heart J* 1995;130:976–86

7. Wong M, Edelstein J, Wollman J, Bond MG. Ultrasonic-pathological comparison of the human arterial wall. Verification of intima-media thickness. *Arterioscler Thromb* 1993;13:482–6

8. Nissen SE, Gurley JC, Grines CL, *et al.* Intravascular ultrasound assessment of lumen size and wall morphology in normal subjects and patients with coronary artery disease. *Circulation* 1991;84:1087–99

9. Mintz GS, Nissen SE, Anderson WD, *et al.* American College of Cardiology Clinical Expert Consensus Document on Standards for Acquisition, Measurement and Reporting of Intravascular Ultrasound Studies (IVUS). A report of the American College of Cardiology Task Force on Clinical Expert Consensus Documents. *J Am Coll Cardiol* 2001;1478–92

10. Di Mario C, Gorge G, Peters R, *et al.* Clinical application and image interpretation in intracoronary ultrasound. Study Group on Intracoronary Imaging of the Working Group of Coronary Circulation and of the Subgroup on Intravascular Ultrasound of the Working Group of Echocardiography of the European Society of Cardiology. *Eur Heart J* 1998;19:207–29

11. Hausmann D, Erbel R, Alibelli-Chemarin MJ, *et al.* The safety of intracoronary ultrasound: a multicenter survey of 2207 examinations. *Circulation* 1995;91:623–30

12. Batkoff BW, Linker DT. Safety of intracoronary ultrasound: data from a Multicenter European Registry. *Cathet Cardiovasc Diagn* 1996;38:238–41

13. Ramasubbu K, Schoenhagen P, Balghith MA, *et al.* Repeated intravascular ultrasound imaging in cardiac transplant recipients does not accelerate transplant coronary artery disease. *J Am Coll Cardiol* 2003;41:1739–43

14. Bruining N, von Birgelen C, Di Mario C, *et al.* Dynamic three-dimensional reconstruction of ICUS images based on an ECG-gated pull-back device. *Computers in Cardiology* 2000;633–6

15. Gil R, Von Birgelen C, Prati F, *et al.* Usefulness of three-dimensional reconstruction for interpretation and quantitative analysis of intracoronary ultrasound

during stent deployment. *Am J Cardiol* 1996;77:761–4

16. Dhawale PJ, Griffin N, Wilson DL, Hodgson JM. Calibrated 3-D reconstruction of intracoronary ultrasound images with cardiac gating and catheter motion compensation. *Computers in Cardiology* 1992;31–4

17. Evans JL, Ng KH, Wiet SG, *et al*. Accurate three-dimensional reconstruction of intravascular ultrasound data. Spatially correct three-dimensional reconstructions. *Circulation* 1996;93:567–76

18. Rosenfield K, Losordo DW, Ramaswamy K, *et al*. Three-dimensional reconstruction of human coronary and peripheral arteries from images recorded during two-dimensional intravascular ultrasound examination. *Circulation* 1991;84:1938–56

19. Klingensmith JD, Schoenhagen P, Tajaddini A, *et al*. Automated three-dimensional assessment of coronary artery anatomy using intravascular ultrasound. *Am Heart J* 2003;145:795–805

20. Linker DT, Kleven A, Gronningsaether A, Yock PG, Angelsen BA. Tissue characterization with intra-arterial ultrasound: special promise and problems. *Int J Card Imaging* 1991;6:255–63

21. Bridal SL, Fornes P, Bruneval P, *et al*. Parametric (integrated backscatter and attenuation) images constructed using backscattered radio frequency signals (25–56 MHz) from human aortae *in vitro*. *Ultrasound Med Biol* 1997;23:215–29

22. Nair A, Kuban BD, Schoenhagen P, Tuzcu EM, Nissen SE, Vince DG. Coronary plaque classification using intravascular ultrasound radiofrequency data analysis. *Circulation* 2002;106:2200–6

23. Kawasaki M, Takatsu H, Noda T, *et al*. Noninvasive quantitative tissue characterization and two-dimensional color-coded map of human atherosclerotic lesions using ultrasound integrated backscatter: comparison between histology and integrated backscatter images. *J Am Coll Cardiol* 2001;38:486–92

24. Takiuchi S, Rakugi H, Honda K, *et al*. Quantitative ultrasonic tissue characterization can identify high-risk atherosclerotic alteration in human carotid arteries. *Circulation* 2000;102:766–70

25. Stahr PM, Hofflinghaus T, Voigtlander T, *et al*. Discrimination of early/intermediate and advanced/complicated coronary plaque types by radiofrequency intravascular ultrasound analysis. *Am J Cardiol* 2002;90:19–23

26. de Korte CL, Pasterkamp G, van der Steen AF, Woutman HA, Bom N. Characterization of plaque components with intravascular ultrasound elastography in human femoral and coronary arteries *in vitro*. *Circulation* 2000;102:617–23

27. Pasterkamp G, Falk E, Woutman H, Borst C. Techniques characterizing the coronary atherosclerotic plaque: influence on clinical decision making? *J Am Coll Cardiol* 2000;36:13–21

28. Alfonso F, Macaya C, Goicolea J, *et al*. Angiographic changes (Dotter effect) produced by intravascular ultrasound imaging before coronary angioplasty. *Am Heart J* 1994;128:244–51

29. Fayad ZA, Fuster V. Clinical imaging of the high-risk or vulnerable atherosclerotic plaque. *Circ Res* 2001;89:305–16

30. Schroeder S, Kopp AF, Baumbach A, *et al*. Noninvasive detection and evaluation of atherosclerotic coronary plaques with multislice computed tomography. *J Am Coll Cardiol* 2001;37:1430–5

31. Fayad ZA, Fuster V, Nikolaou K, Becker C. Computed tomography and magnetic resonance imaging for noninvasive coronary angiography and plaque imaging: current and potential future concepts. *Circulation* 2002;106:2026–34

32. St Goar FG, Pinto FJ, Alderman EL, Fitzgerald PJ, Stadius ML, Popp RL. Intravascular ultrasound imaging of angiographically normal coronary arteries: an *in vivo* comparison with quantitative angiography. *J Am Coll Cardiol* 1991;18:952–8

33. Gussenhoven EJ, Essed CE, Lancee CT, *et al*. Arterial wall characteristics determined by intravascular ultrasound imaging: an *in vitro* study. *J Am Coll Cardiol* 1989;14:947–52

34. Potkin BN, Bartorelli AL, Gessert JM, *et al*. Coronary artery imaging with intravascular high-frequency ultrasound. *Circulation* 1990;81:1575–85

35. Nishimura RA, Edwards WD, Warnes CA, *et al*. Intravascular ultrasound imaging: *in vitro* validation and pathologic correlation. *J Am Coll Cardiol* 1990;16:145–54

36. Fitzgerald PJ, St. Goar FG, Connolly AJ, *et al*. Intravascular ultrasound imaging of coronary arteries. Is three layers the norm? *Circulation* 1992;86:154–8

37. Fitzgerald PJ, Yock C, Yock PG. Orientation of intracoronary ultrasonography: looking beyond the artery. *J Am Soc Echocardiogr* 1998;11:13–19

38. Oesterle SN, Reifart N, Hauptmann E, *et al.* Percutaneous *in situ* coronary venous arterialization: report of the first human catheter-based coronary artery bypass. *Circulation* 2001;103:2539–43

39. Stary HC. Evolution and progression of atherosclerotic lesions in coronary arteries of children and young adults. *Arteriosclerosis* 1989;9(Suppl I):I-19-32

40. Kimura BJ, Russo RJ, Bhargava V, McDaniel MB, Peterson KL, DeMaria AN. Atheroma morphology and distribution in proximal left anterior descending coronary artery: *in vivo* observations. *J Am Coll Cardiol* 1996;27:825–31

41. Badak O, Schoenhagen P, Tsunoda T, *et al.* Characteristics of atherosclerotic plaque distribution in coronary artery bifurcations. An intravascular ultrasound analysis. *Coron Artery Dis* 2003;14:309–16

42. Grottum P, Svindland A, Walloe L. Localization of atherosclerotic lesions in the bifurcation of the main left coronary artery. *Atherosclerosis* 1983;47:55–62

43. Fox B, James K, Morgan B, Seed A. Distribution of fatty and fibrous plaques in young human coronary arteries. *Atherosclerosis* 1982;41:337–47

44. Glagov S, Zarins C, Giddens DP, Ku DN. Hemodynamics and atherosclerosis. *Arch Pathol Lab Med* 1988;112:1018–31

45. ten Hoff H, Korbijn A, Smith TH, *et al.* Imaging artifacts in mechanically driven ultrasound catheters. *Int J Card Imaging* 1989;4:195–9

46. Ge J, Erbel R, Gerber T, *et al.* Intravascular ultrasound imaging of angiographically normal coronary arteries: a prospective study *in vivo*. *Br Heart J* 1994;71:572–8

47. Tsutsui H, Schoenhagen P, Crowe TD, *et al.* Influence of coronary pulsation on volumetric intravascular ultrasound measurements performed without ECG-gating. Validation in vessel segments with minimal disease. *Int J Cardiovascular Imaging* 2003;19:51–7

48. Di Mario C, Madretsma S, Linker D, *et al.* The angle of incidence of the ultrasonic beam: a critical factor for the image quality in intravascular ultrasonography. *Am Heart J* 1993;125:442–8

49. Mintz GS, Douek P, Pichard AD, *et al.* Target lesion calcification in coronary artery disease: an intravascular ultrasound study. *J Am Coll Cardiol* 1992;20:1149–55

50. Tuzcu EM, Berkalp B, De Franco AC, *et al.* The dilemma of diagnosing coronary calcification: angiography versus intravascular ultrasound. *J Am Coll Cardiol* 1996;27:832–8

51. Tobis JM, Mallery JA, Gessert J, *et al.* Intravascular ultrasound cross-sectional arterial imaging before and after balloon angioplasty *in vitro*. *Circulation* 1989;80:873–82

52. Honye J, Mahon DJ, Jain A, *et al.* Morphological effects of coronary balloon angioplasty *in vivo* assessed by intravascular ultrasound imaging. *Circulation* 1992;85:1012–25

53. Waller BF. 'Crackers, breakers, stretchers, drillers, scrapers, shavers, burners, welders, and melters': the future treatment of atherosclerotic coronary artery disease? A clinical-morphologic assessment. *J Am Coll Cardiol* 1989;13:969–7

54. Moreno PR, Purushothaman R, Fuster V, O'Connor WN. Intimomedial interface damage and adventitial inflammation is increased beneath disrupted atherosclerosis in the aorta. Implications for plaque vulnerability. *Circulation* 2002;105:2502–9

55. Glagov S, Weisenberg E, Zarins CK, Stankunavicius R, Kolettis GJ. Compensatory enlargement of human atherosclerotic coronary arteries. *N Engl J Med* 1987;316:1371–5

56. Schoenhagen P, Ziada KM, Vince DG, Nissen, SE, Tuzcu EM. Arterial remodeling and coronary artery disease. The concept of 'dilated' versus 'obstructive' coronary atherosclerosis. *J Am Coll Cardiol* 2001;38:297–306

57. Hermiller JB, Tenaglia AN, Kisslo KB, *et al. In vivo* validation of compensatory enlargement of atherosclerotic coronary arteries. *Am J Cardiol* 1993;71:665–8

58. Losordo DW, Rosenfield K, Kaufman J, Pieczek A, Isner JM. Focal compensatory enlargement of human arteries in response to progressive atherosclerosis. *In vivo* documentation using intravascular ultrasound. *Circulation* 1994;89:2570–7

59. Pasterkamp G, Wensing PJ, Post MJ, Hillen B, Mali WP, Borst C. Paradoxical arterial wall shrinkage may contribute to luminal narrowing of human atherosclerotic femoral arteries. *Circulation* 1995;91:1444–9

60. Mintz GS, Kent KM, Pichard AD, *et al.* Contribution of inadequate arterial remodeling to the development of focal coronary artery stenoses: an intravascular ultrasound study. *Circulation* 1997;95:1791–8

61. Nishioka T, Luo H, Eigler NL, Berglund H, Kim CJ, Siegel RJ. Contribution of inadequate compensatory enlargement to development of human coronary artery stenosis: an *in vivo* intravascular ultrasound study. *J Am Coll Cardiol* 1996;27:1571–6

62. Mintz GS, Popma JJ, Pichard AD, *et al*. Arterial remodeling after coronary angioplasty: a serial intravascular ultrasound study. *Circulation* 1996;94:35–43

63. Kimura T, Kaburagi S, Tamura T, *et al*. Remodeling of human coronary arteries undergoing coronary angioplasty or atherectomy. *Circulation* 1997;96:475–83

64. Schoenhagen P, Ziada K, Kapadia SR, Crowe TD, Nissen SE, Tuzcu EM. Extent and direction of arterial remodeling in stable versus unstable coronary syndromes: an intravascular ultrasound study. *Circulation* 2000;101:598–603

65. Pasterkamp G, Schoneveld AH, van der Wal AC, *et al*. Relation of arterial geometry to luminal narrowing and histologic markers for plaque vulnerability: the remodeling paradox. *J Am Coll Cardiol* 1998;32:655–62

66. Goldberg SL, Colombo A, Nakamura S, Almagor Y, Maiello L, Tobis JM. Benefit of intracoronary ultrasound in the deployment of Palmaz–Schats stents. *J Am Coll Cardiol* 1994;24:996–1003

67. Nakamura S, Colombo A, Gaglione A, *et al*. Intracoronary ultrasound observations during stent implantation. *Circulation* 1994;89:2026–34

68. Nissen SE. Application of intravascular ultrasound to characterize coronary artery disease and assess the progression or regression of atherosclerosis. *Am J Cardiol* 2002;89:24B–31B

69. Schoenhagen P, Nissen SE. Coronary atherosclerotic disease burden: an emerging endpoint in progression/regression studies using intravascular ultrasound. *Curr Drug Targets Cardiovasc Haematol Disord* 2003;3:218–26

70. von Birgelen C, de Vrey EA, Mintz GS, *et al*. ECG-gated three-dimensional intravascular ultrasound: feasibility and reproducibility of the automated analysis of coronary lumen and atherosclerotic plaque dimensions in humans. *Circulation* 1997;96:2944–52

71. Bruining N, von Birgelen C, de Feyter PJ, *et al*. ECG-gated versus nongated three-dimensional intracoronary ultrasound analysis: implications for volumetric measurements. *Cathet Cardiovasc Diagn* 1998;43:254–60

72. Mehran R, Mintz GS, Hong MK, *et al*. Validation of the in vivo intravascular ultrasound measurement of in-stent neointimal hyperplasia volumes. *J Am Coll Cardiol* 1998;32:794–9

73. Prati F, Di Mario C, Moussa I, *et al*. In-stent neointimal proliferation correlates with the amount of residual plaque burden outside the stent: an intravascular ultrasound study. *Circulation* 1999;99:1011–14

74. Topol EJ, Nissen SE. Our preoccupation with coronary luminology: the dissociation between clinical and angiographic findings in ischemic heart disease. *Circulation* 1995;92:2333–42

75. Mintz GS, Painter JA, Pichard AD, *et al*. Atherosclerosis in angiographically 'normal' coronary artery reference segments: an intravascular ultrasound study with clinical correlations. *J Am Coll Cardiol* 1995;25:1479–85

76. Palmer ND, Northridge D, Lessells A, *et al*. *In vitro* analysis of coronary atheromatous lesions by intravascular ultrasound; reproducibility and histological correlation of lesion morphology. *Eur Heart J* 1999;20:1701–6

77. Peters RJ, Kok WE, Havenith MG, *et al*. Histopathologic validation of intracoronary ultrasound imaging. *J Am Soc Echocardiogr* 1994;7:230–41

78. Lockwood GR, Ryan LK, Gotlieb AI, *et al*. *In vitro* high resolution intravascular imaging in muscular and elastic arteries. *J Am Coll Cardiol* 1992;20:153–60

79. Metz JA, Yock PG, Fitzgerald PJ. Intravascular ultrasound: basic interpretation. *Cardiol Clin* 1997;15:1–15

80. Schmermund A, Erbel R. Unstable coronary plaque and its relation to coronary calcium. *Circulation* 2001;104:1682–7

81. Schoenhagen P, Tuzcu EM. Coronary artery calcification and end stage renal disease. Vascular biology and clinical implications. *CCJM* 2002;69(Suppl 3):S12–20

82. Siegel RJ, Ariani M, Fishbein MC, *et al*. Histopathologic validation of angioscopy and intravascular ultrasound. *Circulation* 1991;84:109–17

83. Chung IM, Gold HK, Schwartz SM, Ikari Y, Reidy MA, Wight TN. Enhanced extracellular matrix accumulation in restenosis of coronary arteries after stent deployment. *J Am Coll Cardiol* 2002;40:2072–81

84. Burke AP, Farb A, Malcom GT, *et al.* Coronary risk factors and plaque morphology in men with coronary disease who died suddenly. *N Engl J Med* 1997;336:1276–82

85. Schoenhagen P, Stone GW, Nissen SE, *et al.* Coronary plaque morphology and frequency of ulceration distant from culprit lesions in patients with unstable and stable presentation. *Arterioscler Thromb Vasc Biol* 2003;July 3 [Epub ahead of print]

86. von Birgelen C, Klinkhart W, Mintz GS, *et al.* Size of emptied plaque cavity following spontaneous rupture is related to coronary dimensions, not the degree of lumen narrowing. A study with intravascular ultrasound *in vivo. Heart* 2000;84:483–8

87. Ge J, Chirillo F, Schwedtmann J, *et al.* Screening of ruptured plaques in patients with coronary artery disease by intravascular ultrasound. *Heart* 1999;81:621–7

88. Hodgson JM, Reddy KG, Suneja R, Nair RN, Lesnefsky EJ, Sheehan HM. Intracoronary ultrasound imaging: correlation of plaque morphology with angiography, clinical syndrome and procedural results in patients undergoing coronary angioplasty. *J Am Coll Cardiol* 1993;21:35–44

89. Rasheed Q, Dhawale PJ, Anderson J, Hodgson JM. Intracoronary ultrasound-defined plaque composition: computer-aided plaque characterization and correlation with histologic samples obtained during directional coronary atherectomy. *Am Heart J* 1995;129:631–7

90. Kearney P, Erbel R, Rupprecht HJ, *et al.* Differences in the morphology of unstable and stable coronary lesions and their impact on the mechanisms of angioplasty. An *in vivo* study with intravascular ultrasound. *Eur Heart J* 1996;17:721–30

91. Bocksch W, Schartl M, Beckmann S, *et al.* Intravascular ultrasound imaging in patients with acute myocardial infarction. *Eur Heart J* 1995;16(Suppl J):46–52

92. Smits PC, Pasterkamp G, de Jaegere PPT, *et al.* Angioscopic complex lesions are predominantly compensatory enlarged: an angioscopic and intracoronary ultrasound study. *Cardiovascular Res* 1999;41:458–64

93. Filardo SD, Scharzacher SP, Lo ST, *et al.* Acute myocardial infarction and vascular remodeling. *Am J Cardiol* 2000;85:760–2

94. Schoenhagen P, Vince DG, Ziada KM, *et al.* Association of arterial expansion (expansive remodeling) of bifurcation lesions determined by intravascular ultrasonography with unstable clinical presentation. *Am J Cardiol* 2001;88:785–7

95. Tanaka A, Kawarabayashi T, Nishibori Y, *et al.* No-reflow phenomenon and lesion morphology in patients with acute myocardial infarction. *Circulation* 2002;105:2148–52

96. Yamagishi M, Terashima M, Awano K, *et al.* Morphology of vulnerable coronary plaque: insights from follow-up of patients examined by intravascular ultrasound before and acute coronary syndrome. *J Am Coll Cardiol* 2000;35:106–11

97. Bentzon JF, Pasterkamp G, Falk E. Expansive remodeling is a response of the plaque-related vessel wall in aortic roots of ApoE-deficient mice: an experiment of nature. *Arterioscler Thromb Vasc Biol* 2003;23:257–62

98. Endo M, Tomizawa Y, Nishida H, *et al.* Angiographic findings and surgical treatments of coronary artery involvement in Takayasu arteritis. *J Thorac Cardiovasc Surg* 2003;125:570–7

99. Erbel R, Ge J, Bockisch A, *et al.* Value of intracoronary ultrasound and Doppler in the differentiation of angiographically normal coronary arteries: a prospective study in patients with angina pectoris. *Eur Heart J* 1996;17:880–9

100. Roberts WC, Jones AA. Quantitation of coronary arterial narrowing at necropsy in sudden coronary death. *Am J Cardiol* 1979;44:39–44

101. Ziada KM, Tuzcu EM, De Franco AC, *et al.* Intravascular ultrasound assessment of the prevalence and causes of angiographic 'haziness' following high-pressure coronary stenting. *Am J Cardiol* 1997;80:116–21

102. Lee DY, Eigler N, Luo H, *et al.* Effect of intracoronary ultrasound imaging on clinical decision making. *Am Heart J* 1995;129:1084–93

103. Mintz GS, Pichard AD, Kovach JA, *et al.* Impact of preintervention intravascular ultrasound imaging on transcatheter treatment strategies in coronary artery disease. *Am J Cardiol* 1994;73:423–30

104. Isner JM, Kishel J, Kent KM. Accuracy of angiographic determination of left main coronary arterial narrowing. *Circulation* 1981;63:1056–61

105. Hermiller JB, Buller CE, Tenaglia AN, *et al.* Unrecognized left main coronary artery disease in patients undergoing interventional procedures. *Am J Cardiol* 1993;71:173–6

106. Iyisoy A, Ziada K, Schoenhagen P, *et al*. Intravascular ultrasound evidence of ostial narrowing in nonatherosclerotic left main coronary arteries. *Am J Cardiol* 2002;90:773–5

107. Stark RP, McGinn AL, Wilson RF. Chest pain in cardiac-transplant recipients: evidence of sensory reinnervation after cardiac transplantation. *N Engl J Med* 1991;324:1791–4

108. Mairesse GH, Marwick TH, Melin JA, *et al*. Use of exercise electrocardiography, technetium-99 m-MIBI perfusion tomography, and two-dimensional echocardiography for coronary disease surveillance in a low-prevalence population of heart transplant recipients. *J Heart Lung Transplant* 1995;14:222–9

109. Smart FW, Ballantyne CM, Cocanougher B, *et al*. Insensitivity of noninvasive tests to detect coronary artery vasculopathy after heart transplant. *Am J Cardiol* 1991;67:243–7

110. Uretsky BF, Murali S, Reddy PS, *et al*. Development of coronary artery disease in cardiac transplant patients receiving immunosuppressive therapy with cyclosporine and prednisone. *Circulation* 1987;76:827–34

111. Gao SZ, Alderman EL, Schroeder JS, *et al*. Accelerated coronary vascular disease in the heart transplant patient: coronary arteriographic findings. *J Am Coll Cardiol* 1988;12:334–40

112. Dressler FA, Miller LW. Necropsy versus angiography: how accurate is angiography? *J Heart Lung Transplant* 1992;11:S56–S59

113. Tuzcu EM, DeFranco AC, Goormastic M, *et al*. Dichotomous pattern of coronary atherosclerosis 1 to 9 years after transplantation: insights from systematic intravascular ultrasound imaging. *J Am Coll Cardiol* 1996;27:839–46

114. Tuzcu EM, Kapadia SR, Tutar E, *et al*. High prevalence of coronary atherosclerosis in asymptomatic teenagers and young adults: evidence from intravascular ultrasound. *Circulation* 2001;103:2705–10

115. Yeung AC, Davis SF, Hauptman PJ, *et al*. Incidence and progression of transplant coronary artery disease over 1 year: results of a multicenter trial with use of intravascular ultrasound: Multicenter Intravascular Ultrasound Transplant Study Group. *J Heart Lung Transplant* 1995;14:S215–20

116. Rickenbacher PR, Pinto F, Chenzbraun A, *et al*. Incidence and severity of transplant coronary artery disease early and up to 15 years after transplantation as detected by intravascular ultrasound. *J Am Coll Cardiol* 1995;25:171–7

117. Pinto FJ, Chenzbraun A, Botas J, *et al*. Feasibility of serial intracoronary ultrasound imaging for assessment of progression of intimal proliferation in cardiac transplant recipients. *Circulation* 1994;90:2348–55

118. Mehra MR, Ventura HO, Stapleton DD, *et al*. Presence of severe intimal thickening by intravascular ultrasonography predicts cardiac events in cardiac allograft vasculopathy. *J Heart Lung Transplant* 1995;14:632–9

119. Wiedermann JG, Wasserman HS, Weinberger JZ. Severe intimal thickening by intravascular ultrasonography predicts early death in cardiac transplant recipients. *Circulation* 1994;90:I-93

120. Rickenbacher PR, Pinto FJ, Lewis NP, *et al*. Prognostic importance of intimal thickness as measured by intracoronary ultrasound after cardiac transplantation. *Circulation* 1995;92:3445–52

121. Tuzcu EM, Hobbs RE, Rincon G, *et al*. Occult and frequent transmission of atherosclerotic coronary disease with cardiac transplantation: insights from intravascular ultrasound. *Circulation* 1995;91:1706–13

122. Kapadia SR, Nissen SE, Ziada KM, *et al*. Development of transplantation vasculopathy and progression of donor-transmitted atherosclerosis: comparison by serial intravascular ultrasound imaging. *Circulation* 1998;98:2672–8

123. Konig A, Theisen K, Klauss V. Intravascular ultrasound for assessment of coronary allograft vasculopathy. *Z Kardiol* 2000;89(Suppl 9):IX/45–9

124. Eisen HJ, Tuzcu EM, Dorent R, *et al*., and RAD B253 Study Group. Everolimus for the prevention of allograft rejection and vasculopathy in cardiac-transplant recipients. *N Engl J Med* 2003;349:847–58

125. Hummel M, Dandel M, Knollmann F, *et al*. Long-term surveillance of heart-transplanted patients: noninvasive monitoring of acute rejection episodes and transplant vasculopathy. *Transplant Proc* 2001;33:3539–42

126. Knollmann FD, Bocksch W, Spiegelsberger S, Hetzer R, Felix R, Hummel M. Electron-beam computed tomography in the assessment of coronary artery disease after heart transplantation. *Circulation* 2000;101:2078–82

127. Dangas G, Mintz GS, Mehran R, *et al*. Preintervention arterial remodeling as an independent predictor of target-lesion revascularization after nonstent coronary intervention. *Circulation* 1999;99:3149–54

170. Fuster V. Elucidation of the role of plaque instability and rupture in acute coronary events. *Am J Cardiol* 1995;76:24–33C

171. Falk E, Shah PK, Fuster V. Coronary plaque disruption. *Circulation* 1995;92:657–71

172. Libby P. Molecular bases of the acute coronary syndromes. *Circulation* 1995;91:2844–50

173. Libby P. Current concepts of the pathogenesis of the acute coronary syndromes. *Circulation* 2001;104:365–72

174. Newby AC, Libby P, van der Wal A. Plaque instability – the real challenge for atherosclerosis research in the next decade? *Cardiovasc Res* 1999;41:321–22

175. Gutstein DE, Fuster V. Pathophysiology and clinical significance of atherosclerotic plaque rupture. *Cardiovascular Research* 1999;41:323–33

176. Ross R. The pathogenesis of atherosclerosis: a perspective for the 1990's. *Nature* 1993;362:801–9

177. Fuster V, Badimon L, Badimon JJ Chesebro JH. The pathogenesis of coronary artery disease and the acute coronary syndromes. I. *N Engl J Med* 1992;326: 242–50

178. Fuster V, Badimon L, Badimon JJ Chesebro JH. The pathogenesis of coronary artery disease and the acute coronary syndromes. II. *N Engl J Med* 1992;326: 310–18

179. Burke AP, Kolodgie FD, Farb A, *et al*. Healed plaque ruptures and sudden coronary death. *Circulation* 2001;103:934–40

180. Williams H, Johnson JL, Carson KGS, Jackson CL. Characteristics of intact and ruptured atherosclerotic plaques in brachiocephalic arteries of apolipoprotein E knockout mice. *Arterioscler Thromb Vasc Biol* 2002;22:788–92

181. Frink RJ. Chronic ulcerated plaques: new insights into the pathogenesis of acute coronary disease. *J Invas Cardiol* 1994;6:173–85

182. Buffon A, Biasucci LM, Liuzzo G, D'Onofrio G, Crea F, Maseri A. Widespread coronary inflammation in unstable angina. *N Engl J Med* 2002;347:5–12

183. Asakura M, Ueda Y, Yamaguchi O, *et al*. Extensive development of vulnerable plaques as a pan-coronary process in patients with myocardial infarction: an angioscopic study. *J Am Coll Cardiol* 2001;37:1284–8

184. Rioufol G, Finet G, Ginon I, *et al*. Multiple atherosclerotic plaque rupture in acute coronary syndrome.

A three-vessel intravascular ultrasound study. *Circulation* 2002;106:804–8

185. Maehara A, Mintz GS, Bui AB, *et al*. Morphologic and angiographic features of coronary plaque rupture detected by intravascular ultrasound. *J Am Coll Cardiol* 2002;40:904–10

186. Schoenhagen P, Tuzcu EM, Ellis SG. Plaque vulnerability, plaque rupture, and acute coronary syndromes. (Multi)-focal manifestation of a systemic disease process. *Circulation* 2002;106:760–2

187. Goldstein JA, Demetriou D, Grines CL, *et al*. Multiple complex coronary plaques in patients with acute myocardial infarction. *N Engl J Med* 2000;343:915–22

188. Pasterkamp G, Schoneveld AH, van der Wal AC, *et al*. Inflammation of the atherosclerotic cap and shoulder of the plaque is a common and locally observed feature in unruptured plaques of femoral and coronary arteries. *Arterioscler Thromb Vasc Biol* 1999;19:54–8

189. Tuzcu EM, Schoenhagen P. Acute coronary syndromes, plaque vulnerability, and carotid artery disease. The changing role of atherosclerosis imaging. *J Am Coll Cardiol* 2003;42:1033–6

190. Burke AP, Kolodgie FD, Farb A, Weber D, Virmani R. Morphological predictors of arterial remodeling in coronary atherosclerosis. *Circulation* 2002;105: 297–303

191. Varnava AM, Mills PG, Davies MJ. Relationship between coronary artery remodeling and plaque vulnerability. *Circulation* 2002;105:939–43

192. Galis ZS, Sukhova GK, Lark MW, Libby P. Increased expression of matrix metalloproteinases and matrix degrading activity in vulnerable regions of human atherosclerotic plaques. *J Clin Invest* 1994;94:2493–503

193. Henney AM, Wakeley PR, Davies MJ, *et al*. Localization of stromelysin gene expression in atherosclerotic plaques by in situ hybridization. *Proc Natl Acad Sci USA* 1991;88:8154–8

194. Nagase H, Woessner JF. Matrix metalloproteinases. *J Biol Chem* 1999;274,31:21491–4

195. Ye S, Humphries S, Henney A. Matrix metalloproteinases: implication in vascular matrix remodeling during atherogenesis. *Clin Sci* 1998;94:103–10

196. Dollery CM, McEwan JR, Henney AM. Matrix metalloproteinases and cardiovascular disease. *Circ Res* 1995;77:863–8

197. Schoenhagen P, Vince DG, Ziada KM, *et al*. Relation of matrix-metalloproteinase 3 found in coronary lesion samples retrieved by directional coronary atherectomy to intravascular ultrasound observations on coronary remodeling. *Am J Cardiol* 2002;89:1354–9

198. Pasterkamp G, Schoneveld AH, Hijnen DJ, *et al*. Atherosclerotic arterial remodeling and the localization of macrophages and matrix metalloproteases 1, 2 and 9 in the human coronary artery. *Atherosclerosis* 2000;150:245–53

199. Brown DL, Hibbs MS, Kearney M, Loushin C, Isner JM. Identification of 92-kD gelatinase in human coronary atherosclerotic lesions. *Circulation* 1995;91:2125–31

200. Hartnell GG, Parnell BM, Pridie RB. Coronary artery ectasia. Its prevalence and clinical significance in 4993 patients. *Br Heart J* 1985;54:392–5

201. Swanton RH, Lea Thomas M, Coltart DJ, Jenkins BS, Webb-Peploe MM, Williams BT. Coronary artery ectasia – a variant of occlusive coronary arteriosclerosis. *Br Heart J* 1978;40:393–400

202. Berkoff HA, Rowe GG. Atherosclerotic ulcerative disease and associated aneurysms of the coronary arteries. *Am Heart J* 1975;90:153–8

203. Small DM, Bond MG, Waugh D, Prack M, Sawyer JK. Physicochemical and histological changes in the arterial wall of nonhuman primates during progression and regression of atherosclerosis. *J Clin Invest* 1984;73:1590–605

204. Lutgens E, Gijbels M, Smook M, *et al*. Transforming growth factor-beta mediates balance between inflammation and fibrosis during plaque progression. *Arterioscler Thromb Vasc Biol* 2002;22:975–82

205. Little WC, Constantinescu M, Applegate RJ, *et al*. Can coronary angiography predict the site of a subsequent myocardial infarction in patients with mild-to-moderate coronary artery disease? *Circulation* 1988;78:1157–66

206. Giroud D, Li JM, Urban P, Meier B, Rutishauser W. Relation of the site of acute myocardial infarction to the most severe coronary arterial stenosis prior to angiography. *Am J Cardiol* 1992;69:729–32

207. Ambrose JA, Tannenbaum MA, Alexopoulos D, *et al*. Angiographic progression of coronary artery disease and the development of myocardial infarction. *J Am Coll Cardiol* 1988;12:56–62

208. Qiao JH, Fishbein MC. The severity of coronary atheroclerosis at sites of plaque rupture with occlusive thrombosis. *J Am Coll Cardiol* 1991;17:1138–42

209. Falk E. Plaque rupture with severe pre-existing stenosis precipitating coronary thrombosis. Characteristics of coronary atherosclerotic plaques underlying fatal occlusive thrombi. *Br Heart J* 1983;50:127–34

210. Horie T, Sekiguchi M, Hirosawa K. Coronary thrombosis in pathogenesis of acute myocardial infarction. *Br Heart J* 1978;40:153–61

211. Davies MJ, Thomas A. Thrombosis and acute coronary artery lesions in sudden cardiac ischemic death. *N Engl J Med* 1984;310:1137–40

212. Strong JP, Malcom GT, McMahan CA, *et al*. Prevalence and extent of atherosclerosis in adolescents and young adults: implications for prevention from pathobiological determinants of atherosclerosis in youth study. *J Am Med Assoc* 1999;281:727–35

213. Schoenhagen P, Magyar WA, Kapadia SR, *et al*. Negative remodeling frequently occurs in mildly stenotic native coronary lesions and is unrelated to plaque size. *J Am Coll Cardiol* 2002;39(Suppl A:246A): Abstr 834–2

214. Schoenhagen P, Tuzcu EM, Stillman AE, *et al*. Non-invasive assessment of plaque morphology and remodeling in mildly stenotic coronary segments: comparison of 16-slice computed tomography and intravascular ultrasound. *Coron Artery Dis* 2003;14:459–62

215. Schoenhagen P, Halliburton SS, Stillman AE, *et al*. Non-invasive imaging of the coronary arteries: current and future role of multi-slice computed tomography (MSCT). *Radiology* 2003;in press

216. Schoenhagen P, Tsunoda T, Kapadia S, *et al*. Independent remodeling pattern of sequential coronary plaques in the same artery. An intravascular ultrasound study. *ATVB* 2003;23:Abstr 77

217. Klingensmith JD, Vince DG, Kuban BD, *et al*. Assessment of coronary compensatory enlargement by three-dimensional intravascular ultrasound. *Int J Cardiac Imaging* 2000;16:87–98

218. Shiran A, Mintz GS, Leiboff B, *et al*. Serial volumetric intravascular ultrasound assessment of arterial remodeling in left main coronary artery disease. *Am J Cardiol* 1999;83:1427–32

219. Schartl M, Bocksch W, Koschyk DH, *et al*. Use of intravascular ultrasound to compare effects of different strategies of lipid-lowering therapy on plaque volume and composition in patients with

coronary artery disease. *Circulation* 2001;104:387–92

220. Tsutsui H, Schoenhagen P, Klingensmith JD, Vince DG, Nissen SE, Tuzcu EM. Regression of a donor atheroma after cardiac transplantation: serial observations with intravascular ultrasound. *Circulation* 2001;104:2874

221. Tsutsui H, Ziada KM, Schoenhagen P, *et al.* Lumen loss in transplant coronary artery disease is a biphasic process involving early intimal thickening and late constrictive remodeling: results from a 5-year serial intravascular ultrasound study. *Circulation* 2001;104:653–7

222. Tsutsui H, Schoenhagen P, Ziada KM, *et al.* Early constriction or expansion of the external elastic membrane area determines the late remodeling response and cumulative lumen loss in transplant vasculopathy: an intravascular ultrasound study with 4-year follow-up. *J Heart Lung Transplant* 2003;22:519–25

223. Takagi T, Yoshida K, Akasaka T, *et al.* Intravascular ultrasound analysis of reduction in progression of coronary narrowing by treatment with pravastatin. *Am J Cardiol* 1997;79:1673–6

224. Matsuzaki M, Hiramori K, Imaizumi T, *et al.* Intravascualar ultrasound evaluation of coronary plaque regression by low density lipoprotein-apheresis in familial hypercholesterolemia. *J Am Coll Cardiol* 2002;40:220–7

225. Cao JJ, Thach C, Manolio TA, *et al.* C-reactive protein, carotid intima-media thickness, and incidence of ischemic stroke in the elderly. The Cardiovascular Health Study. *Circulation* 2003;108:166–70

226. Kim WY, Stuber M, Börnert P, *et al.* Three-dimensional black-blood cardiac magnetic resonance coronary vessel wall imaging detects positive arterial remodeling in patients with nonsignificant coronary artery disease. *Circulation* 2002;106:296–9

227. Nieman K, Cademartiri F, Lemos PA, *et al.* Reliable noninvasive coronary angiography with fast sub-millimeter multislice spiral computed tomography. *Circulation* 2002;106:2051–4

228. Ropers D, Baum U, Pohle K, *et al.* Detection of coronary artery stenoses with thin-slice multi-detector row spiral computed tomography and multi-planar reconstruction. *Circulation* 2003;107:664–6

Index